SPINE
SURGERY
A PRACTICAL ATLAS

NOTICE

Medicine is an ever-changing science. As new research and clinical experience broaden our knowledge, changes in treatment and drug therapy are required. The editors and the publisher of this work have checked with sources believed to be reliable in their efforts to provide information that is complete and generally in accord with the standards accepted at the time of publication. However, in view of the possibility of human error or changes in medical sciences, neither the editors nor the publisher nor any other party who has been involved in the preparation or publication of this work warrants that the information contained herein is in every respect accurate or complete, and they disclaim all responsibility for any errors or omissions or for the results obtained from use of such information contained in this work. Readers are encouraged to confirm the information contained herein with other sources. For example and in particular, readers are advised to check the product information sheet included in the package of each drug they plan to administer to be certain that the information contained in this work is accurate and that changes have not been made in the recommended dose or in the contraindications for administration. This recommendation is of particular importance in connection with new or infrequently used drugs.

SPINE
SURGERY
A PRACTICAL ATLAS

F. Todd Wetzel, M.D.

Associate Professor of Surgery
Section of Orthopaedic Surgery & Rehabilitation
Anesthesia and Critical Care
Chairman, Division of Surgery
Louis A. Weiss Hospital/University of Chicago Hospitals
Chicago, Illinois

Edward Nathaniel Hanley, Jr., M.D.

Chairman, Department of Orthopaedics
Vice President, Medical Education & Research
Carolinas Medical Center
Charlotte, North Carolina

With illustrations by
Pat Thomas, C.M.I., F.A.M.I., and Christa Wellman, M.A.M.S,
Oak Park, Illinois

McGRAW-HILL
MEDICAL PUBLISHING DIVISION

New York   Chicago   San Francisco   Lisbon   London   Madrid   Mexico City   Milan
New Delhi   San Juan   Seoul   Singapore   Sydney   Toronto

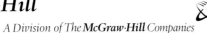

McGraw-Hill

A Division of The McGraw·Hill Companies

SPINE SURGERY: A PRACTICAL ATLAS
Copyright © 2002 by **The McGraw-Hill Companies,** Inc. All rights reserved.
Printed in Hong Kong. Except as permitted under the United States Copyright
Act of 1976, no part of this publication may be reproduced or distributed in
any form or by any means, or stored in a data base or retrieval system, with-
out the prior written permission of the publisher.

1 2 3 4 5 6 7 8 9 0 IMAIMA 0 9 8 7 6 5 4 3 2

ISBN 0-8385-8617-1

This book was set in Optima at Imago (USA).
The editors were Darlene Cooke, Susan Noujaim, Nicky Panton,
   and Lynn M. Ridings.
The production supervisor was Catherine H. Saggese.
The text designer was Marsha Cohen/Parallelogram Graphics.
The cover designer was Aimee Nordin.
The index was prepared by Barbara Littlewood.

Imago was printer and binder.

This book is printed on acid-free paper.

Library of Congress Cataloging-in-Publication Data
Wetzel, F. Todd.
   Spine surgery: a practical atlas / F. Todd Wetzel, Edward Nathaniel
Hanley, Jr.
      p. ; cm.
   Includes bibliographical references and index.
   ISBN 0-8385-8617-1 (alk. paper)
     1. Spine—Surgery—Atlases. I. Hanley, Edward N. II. Title.
   [DNLM: 1. Spine—surgery—Atlases. WE 17 W544s 2002]
RD768 .W4285 2002
617.5′6059—dc21   2001031258

CONTENTS

PART II

THORACIC SPINE / 89

PREFACE

The core of medicine in general, and surgery in particular, is changing rapidly. As physicians, a challenge that faces us all is to educate our peers and the generations to come. Unfortunately, in a society that is increasingly preoccupied with economic efficiency and rapid data collection, this challenge has become even greater. As educational institutions are required to compete with more clinically oriented private institutions, graduate and postgraduate education will clearly suffer. Thus, the availability of understandable and concise reference materials is of paramount importance—perhaps more so now than at any time in the past.

It is the intention of the authors to provide a concise summary of current indications, techniques and outcomes for a variety of spinal surgical procedures. As one of the authors remarked, "This work is intended to be the meat of spine surgery." It is intended to be used as an elective reference work as well as a "night before" or "morning of" book. While the work was initially intended for physicians in training, the applicability may be even broader.

It is our hope that this book will provide a concise reference for busy clinicians. The book is not intended to be a definitive or detailed work on any of the procedures, indications, techniques or outcomes mentioned. In this sense, it should fulfill the paramount requirement for any educational material of substance—to stimulate further reading on the subject in question.

F. Todd Wetzel, M.D.
Edward N. Hanley, Jr., M.D.

ACKNOWLEDGMENTS

This book originally began as the brainchild of Edward Wickland at a meeting of the American Academy of Orthopaedic Surgeons. The initial concept, a detailed multi-volume atlas, evolved to the current format. Given the variety of such works on spinal disorders and their care, the practical utility of a more compact and portable reference work became apparent, and from this concept grew *Spine Surgery: A Practical Atlas.*

Aside from Mr. Wickland, the authors are indebted to Michael Medina for his initial management and persistent development of the project. Most of all, the authors are indebted to Pat Thomas and Christa Wellman for their wonderful illustrations. The patience and occasional frustration that these gifted illustrators displayed was to their credit as they attempted to alter the minutiae of their art to the preordained concepts of the authors. Finally, a monumental debt of gratitude is owed to Lynn M. Ridings, who not only served as transcriptionist, critic and editor, but also as motivator, and, in the final analysis, advocate. That Lynn completed the work with her sanity, is a minor miracle. The authors remain grateful not only for this, but for her not inconsiderable talents as well.

Any errors in the manuscript, stylistic or content, are the responsibility of the authors. The content of the text was written after detailed discussions and references to contemporary literature. Obviously, these are somewhat subject to interpretations and prejudices that we frankly acknowledge.

While no work can be free of controversial statements in the current atmosphere in spine surgery, we hope that the offenses to various points of view will be minimal and accepted with the spirit of academic difference.

PART I

LUMBAR SPINE

1

HERNIATED LUMBAR DISK

- ## LAMINOTOMY – DISKECTOMY
- ## DISK EXCISION – FAR LATERAL

- ## LAMINOTOMY–DISKECTOMY

SUMMARY

Symptomatic lumbar disk herniation resulting in sciatica occurs in approximately 2% of the adult population. Ninety percent of patients improve with nonoperative care within 6 to 12 weeks of the onset of symptoms. One exception is the cauda equina syndrome, an acute surgical emergency characterized by multiple nerve root involvement, saddle anesthesia, and urinary retention. In the absence of the cauda equina syndrome, progressive neurologic deterioration, or intolerable pain, nonoperative care is the rule. In those individuals who are refractory to nonoperative care and remain persistently symptomatic after 6 to 12 weeks, laminotomy and diskectomy might be considered. In appropriately selected patients, the success rate of laminotomy with diskectomy should approach 100% in terms of pain relief and functional improvement.

PRESENTATION

In posterior and posterolateral disk prolapses, referred neurogenic pain (sciatica) typically radiates distal to the knee. The distribution of this pain differs according to the nerve roots involved. Ninety percent of disk prolapses involve the L_{4-5} and $L_5–S_1$ segments. Disk prolapse involving the L_{4-5} segment results in symptoms from L_5 root compression. Pain radiates posterolaterally to the dorsum of the foot and the first web space. Weakness of the extensor hallucis longus may be noted. Sensation is frequently diminished in the lateral aspect of the calf. Posterolateral L_5–S_1 disk prolapse involves the S_1 nerve root. The pain radiates posteriorly to the heel. Sensation is altered in this area. The ankle jerk is diminished or absent and weakness might be noted in the gastrocnemius soleus group. More rostral disk herniations, e.g., L_{3-4}, might involve the L_4 nerve root, with pain radiating down the medial aspect of the leg, and weakness of the tibialis anterior. Sensation is altered on the medial leg and the knee-jerk reflex is diminished.

The hallmark of acute disk prolapse and sciatica is the presence of nerve root tension signs. The femoral stretch reproduces pain in the distribution of the involved nerve root in neural compression syndromes involving the L_3 or L_4 nerve roots. The straight-leg raising maneuver of Lasègue is positive, reproducing sciatic pain, when the L_5 or S_1 nerve roots are involved.

The acute cauda equina syndrome is caused by a large central disk prolapse involving multiple nerve roots. The triad of bilateral sciatica, saddle anesthesia, and urinary retention is diagnostic. Physical examination shows weakness, sensory dysesthesias, or reflex changes at many levels; straight-leg raising maneuvers will invariably be positive. The treatment includes immediate imaging in the form of myelography or Magnetic Resonance Imaging (MRI) and immediate surgical decompression. Even with prompt surgical decompression, 30% to 40% will have residual genitourinary or gastrointestinal dysfunction. The sentinel symptom is urinary retention, not incontinence. Overflow incontinence may occur only as a consequence of cauda equina syndrome when it is due to a distended, neurogenic bladder.

NONOPERATIVE CARE

Randomized prospective data have confirmed the efficacy of a brief period of bed rest (less than 48 hours), the use of nonsteroidal anti-inflammatory agents, and active physical therapy as tolerated in the nonoperative treatment of acute disk prolapse. The efficacy of oral or epidural steroids has not been convincingly demonstrated in randomized prospective studies. Likewise, passive physical therapy (e.g., modalities) has not been shown to be of any benefit; manipulation in particular should be avoided. The use of Transcutaneous Electrical Nerve Stimulation (TENS) is controversial. It has been shown to be of benefit in chronic neuropathic pain syndromes, but its utility in acute radiculopathy secondary to lumbar disk prolapse is unproven.

DIAGNOSTIC STUDIES

In cases of persistent symptomatology after 6 to 12 weeks of appropriate conservative care, the imaging modality of choice is MRI. In the patient without previous surgery, gadolinium enhancement is not necessary. In cases of so-called hard disks (disk prolapse associated with ossification or calcification), myelography followed by postmyelographic Computed Tomography (CT) may be beneficial because of the superior definition of bony architecture.

The use of Electromyography and Nerve Conduction Velocity (EMG/NCV) is controversial. Various investigators have shown that the likelihood of isolating a specific nerve root without motor findings is low. Overall, EMG/NCV provides little information in addition to that provided by a comprehensive neurologic examination.

PROCEDURE

LAMINOTOMY – DISKECTOMY (FIG. 1–1)

Laminotomy with diskectomy is performed most frequently under general anesthesia.

POSITIONING

The patient is placed prone, with the abdomen hanging free, usually in a knee-to-chest configuration (Fig. 1–1A). This configuration reverses lumbar lordosis and improves access to the interlaminar space. The appropriate level is localized by an x-ray.

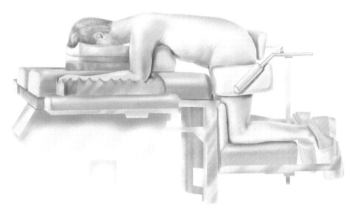

FIGURE 1–1A

HERNIATED DISK LAMINOTOMY–DISKECTOMY (L$_{4-5}$) POSITIONING. The patient is positioned prone in a standard knee-to-chest configuration, with the abdomen hanging free.

TECHNIQUE

To minimize soft tissue morbidity, the use of an operating microscope, surgical loupes, or endoscopic visualization has increased significantly. With these techniques, the incision can be kept small (Fig. 1–1B). In general, the incision for single-level laminotomy/diskectomy should be 3 to 5 cm. Before the incision, the skin may be anesthetized with 1% lidocaine and epinephrine at the discretion of the surgeon.

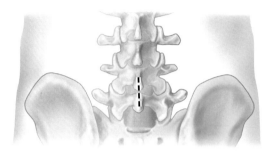

FIGURE 1–1B

The skin is incised in the midline from the spinous process of L$_4$ to L$_5$ (3 to 5 cm).

The skin is incised and self-retaining retractors are inserted. After appropriate hemostasis, dissection is carried through the subcutaneous fat to the lumbar dorsal fascia. The midline is easily visualized by palpating the groove over the spinous processes. This fascia is then divided on the side of the disk prolapse; a lateral spinal dissection then follows, with reflection of the muscles to the level of the facets. Care should be taken to spare the facet capsule.

A self-retaining retractor is then inserted and soft tissue removed from the interspace (Fig. 1–1C). The ligamentum flavum is gently dissected free and removed with

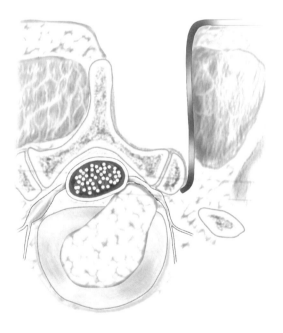

FIGURE 1-1C

On axial projection, the L$_5$ root is compressed by the posterolateral disk herniation.

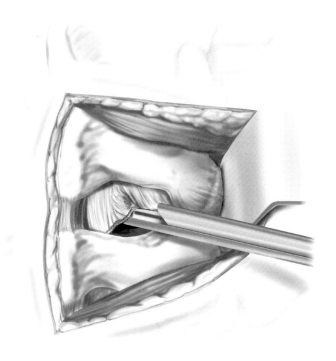

FIGURE 1-1D

The ligamentum flavum is removed by sharp and blunt dissection. Minimal bony resection is required.

a Kerrison rongeur (Fig. 1–1D). A laminotomy is then performed, with partial facetectomy if needed. The ligamentous fibers overlying the lumbar nerve root and defining the foraminal entry zone should be removed with a Kerrison rongeur to facilitate nerve root visualization laterally. After hemostasis with bipolar electrocautery, the affected nerve root is swept medially and the disk fragment visualized. The nerve root *must* be visualized or mobilized to prevent injury; in cases of an adherent root, the nerve trunk might be confused with disk tissue if mobilization is not done. The disk is nearly always more central to the nerve trunk. The annulus is then incised and the fragment removed (Fig. 1–1E). The nerve should then be inspected rostrally, caudally, and medially to be certain that no residual disk compression remains.

The wound is then closed in appropriate layers to include fascia, subcutaneous soft tissues, and skin.

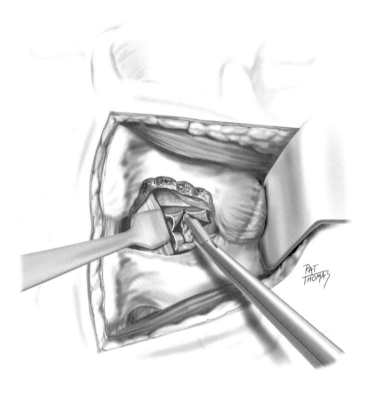

FIGURE 1-1E

A nerve root retractor pulls the shoulder of the L$_5$ root medially. A cruciate incision is made over the disk prolapse. This material is removed with a pituitary rongeur. The disk is always anterior to the exiting nerve root that must be identified and protected during diskectomy.

POSTOPERATIVE CARE

No postoperative orthosis is required. The patient is mobilized as quickly as possible after surgery and instructed in gentle stretching exercises to facilitate neural mobility. These consist of sitting and seated straight-leg raising.

OUTCOMES

A prompt recovery after successful diskectomy for sciatica is the rule, with reports in the literature of many patients returning to unrestricted vocational activities within several weeks of the procedure. Overall, the success rate for pain relief approaches 100% when the following conditions are met: (1) positive root tension signs, (2) pain in the distribution of a nerve root, (3) motor or sensory findings in the appropriate myotome or dermatome, and (4) an objective imaging modality (MRI/CT myelography) precisely concordant with the clinical picture.

COMPLICATIONS

Complications with this procedure are rare but can include transient sensory dysesthesias or recurrent disk prolapse. In general, the risk of recurrent disk herniation (4% to 18%) does not appear to be influenced by the amount of disk resected.

• DISK EXCISION – FAR LATERAL

SUMMARY

Far lateral disk prolapse (intraforaminal) is less common than posterolateral prolapse. It generally occurs in older patients (60 to 70 years) and commonly involves L_3 or L_4 nerve roots.

PRESENTATION AND NONOPERATIVE CARE

Patients present with symptoms in the L_3 or L_4 nerve root distributions. Due to the extremely lateral location of the disk prolapse, L_{3-4} disk prolapse compresses the L_3, not L_4, nerve root, as is the case with the more common posterolateral L_{3-4} prolapse. Likewise, a far lateral disk prolapse at L_{4-5} results in compression of the L_4 nerve root. Appropriate nonoperative care is identical to that for the more common posterolateral disk prolapse.

DIAGNOSTIC STUDIES

MRI and CT myelography have led to an increase in the diagnosis of this entity. Arguably, the most specific study to diagnose this is an intradiskal injection (diskography) followed by postdiskographic CT. In a series of studies comparing this modality with MRI, CT, myelography, and CT myelography, diskography with CT was the most sensitive and specific for diagnosing far lateral disk herniations, provided the herniation remains in continuity with the remainder of the disk (contained prolapse).

PROCEDURE

DISK EXCISION – FAR LATERAL (FIG. 1–2)

POSITIONING

The patient is placed prone, with the abdomen hanging free, usually in a knee-to-chest configuration (Fig. 1–2A). This reverses lumbar lordosis and improves access to the interlaminar space. The appropriate level is localized by x-ray.

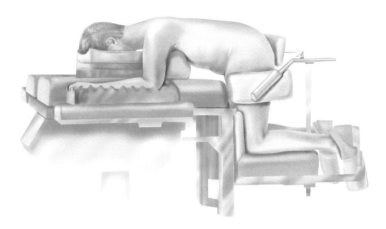

FIGURE 1–2A

FAR LATERAL DISK EXCISION. The patient is positioned prone in a standard knee-to-chest configuration, with the abdomen hanging free.

TECHNIQUE

An incision is made lateral to the midline approximating the lateral line of the facets at the origin of the transverse processes (Fig. 1–2B). Dissection is carried bluntly down to the intertransverse ligament, with exposure of the appropriate transverse processes. A self-retaining retractor is inserted (Fig. 1–2C). The intertransverse membrane is then divided and the nerve root visualized. The nerve runs diagonally from a superomedial to an inferolateral direction (Fig. 1–2D). The nerve is isolated and retracted caudally; dissection is then carried medially toward the intervertebral foramen. A Kerrison rongeur is typically required to remove a portion of the lateral facet. When this is accomplished and the nerve root is retracted rostrally, the disk herniation is immediately apparent. The herniation is *anterior* to the root. The membrane overlying it is incised and the fragment removed (Fig. 1–2E).

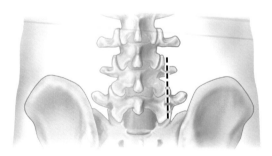

FIGURE 1–2B

The incision is made two to three fingerbreadths lateral to the midline, in this instance, from the L_{3-4} facet to the L_{4-5} facet.

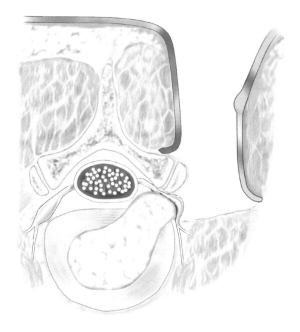

FIGURE 1-2C

The extent of retraction required lateral to the facet is evident in the axial projection. The far lateral L_{4-5} disk prolapse compresses the L_4 nerve root.

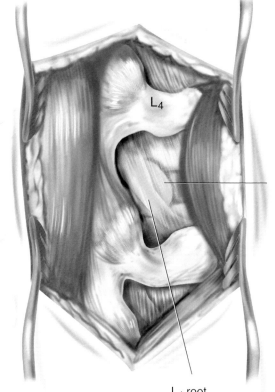

L_4

Herniated disk

L_4 root
beneath
transverse
membrane

FIGURE 1-2D

The intertransverse membrane is visualized. Deep to the membrane, the far lateral disk prolapse at L_{4-5} displaces the L_4 root. Depending on the prolapse, the root might be medial or lateral to the disk herniation.

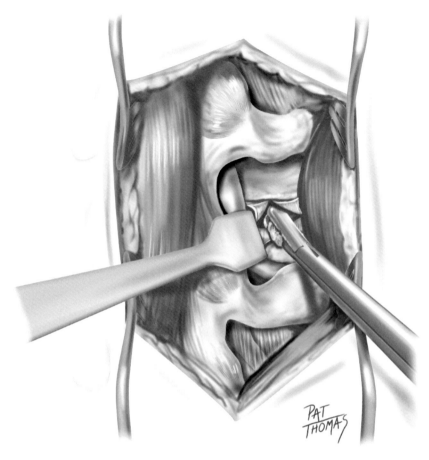

FIGURE 1-2E

The L$_4$ root is retracted caudally with a Love retractor. A cruciate incision is made over the disk prolapse. A pituitary rongeur is used to remove disk material.

The wound is then closed in layers to include fascia, subcutaneous tissue, and skin.

POSTOPERATIVE CARE

The patient is mobilized as quickly as possible after surgery and instructed in gentle exercises to facilitate neural mobility. Exercises consist of sitting and seated straight-leg raising.

OUTCOMES

Most investigators have reported a 70% success rate in terms of pain relief and improved function with the lateral extraforaminal disk herniation procedure. The risk of recurrent disk herniation is unknown with this procedure.

COMPLICATIONS

Transient sensory changes have been reported as a risk of this procedure. In addition, the likelihood of proximal nerve root injury is greater if the exit zone of the neural foramen is not well visualized. Typically, if a partial nerve root injury (rhizotomy) occurs as a result of this procedure, there is little or no intraoperative leakage of cerebrospinal fluid because the injury is postganglionic. Persistent postoperative dysesthesias lasting longer than 18 months, most frequently burning in character, suggest root injury.

2

LUMBAR SPINAL STENOSIS

- ## DECOMPRESSIVE LAMINECTOMY

- ## DECOMPRESSIVE LAMINECTOMY

SUMMARY

The exact incidence of lumbar spinal stenosis resulting in symptomatic neurogenic claudication is unknown. It is, however, a disease associated with degenerative change in the spine and circumferential narrowing of the central spinal canal or neuroforaminal stenosis. This typically occurs in people older than 60 years.

PRESENTATION

In lateral recess stenosis, the patient presents with unilateral or bilateral lower extremity pain that is related to activities or postures that diminish foraminal dimensions (extension). The patient might complain of pain or numbness radiating down the extremity when moving from a flexed to an extended position. Onset of symptoms may be immediate when the patient stands. Symptoms may or may not worsen with ambulation.

In central stenosis, the chief complaint is neurogenic claudication: bilateral or unilateral lower extremity symptoms described as heaviness, numbness, or aching. Those symptoms are related to ambulation. Any activity that results in spinal flexion, thus increasing central and neuroforaminal dimensions, tends to diminish the severity of symptoms; e.g., a patient may note that ambulatory tolerance is increased when walking in a flexed position while bent over a shopping cart. In addition, these patients cannot sleep in a prone position because of provocation of symptoms. This must be differentiated from vascular claudication, which also presents as activity-related lower extremity symptoms. The patient with vascular claudication simply must stop walking for the symptoms to abate; the patient with neurogenic claudication must change positions: sitting down, flexing the trunk, or leaning.

Findings on physical examination are non-specific. The neurologic examination may be normal or there may be signs of single or multiple root dysfunction.

NONOPERATIVE CARE

A trial of nonsteroidal anti-inflammatory medications or flexion-based physical therapy might be beneficial, but firm evidence for this in the literature is lacking. Likewise, there are anecdotal reports suggesting epidural steroids are beneficial in the control of symptoms resulting from lumbar spinal stenosis. There are no randomized prospective studies to support or refute that contention.

DIAGNOSTIC STUDIES

The anatomic diagnosis of lumbar spinal stenosis is made by MRI or CT myelography. Neither modality has been shown to be superior to the other. Whereas MRI is not invasive and provides information concerning the state of disk hydration and marrow changes, myelography followed by CT is superior for delineation of bony detail. Other studies such as EMG/NCV, somatosensory evoked potential monitoring, or technetium scanning have proven to be of no value in the diagnostic evaluation of these conditions.

PROCEDURE

DECOMPRESSIVE LAMINECTOMY (FIG. 2–1)

In the patient who does not respond to conservative care or presents with persistent symptomatology, the procedure of choice is decompressive laminectomy.

POSITIONING

After induction of general endotracheal anesthesia, the patient is placed prone in a knee-to-chest position or an attitude of mild flexion (Fig. 2–1A). A midline incision is made and the dissection is carried down to the levels in question (Fig. 2–1B). Paraspinous muscles are stripped laterally to the facets and a self-retaining retractor is inserted (Fig. 2–1C).

Supraspinous and intraspinous ligaments are then removed with a large rongeur and spinous processes are trimmed. The canal is entered laterally by elevation of the ligamentum flavum or in the midline after removal of the spinous processes and supraspinous and intraspinous ligaments and thinning the remaining laminae with a high-speed burr (Fig. 2–1D). The decompression should include bony elements as

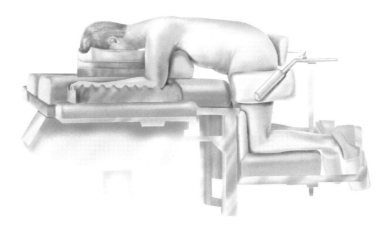

FIGURE 2–1A

DECOMPRESSIVE LAMINECTOMY POSITIONING. The patient may be positioned prone in a knee-to-chest position or an attitude of mild flexion. The knee-to-chest position is shown.

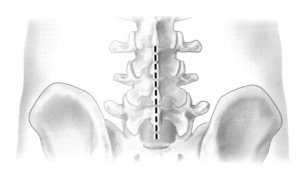

FIGURE 2–1B

A midline incision is made from L_{2-3} to L_5-S_1 to decompress the L_{3-4} and L_{4-5} segments.

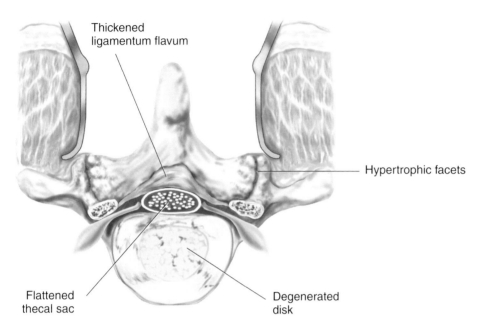

Thickened
ligamentum flavum

Hypertrophic facets

Flattened
thecal sac

Degenerated
disk

FIGURE 2-1C

The circumferential nature of spinal stenosis is evident in the axial plane. Note infolding of the ligamentum flavum, facet hypertrophy, and disk degeneration, which result in flattening and attenuation of the thecal sac.

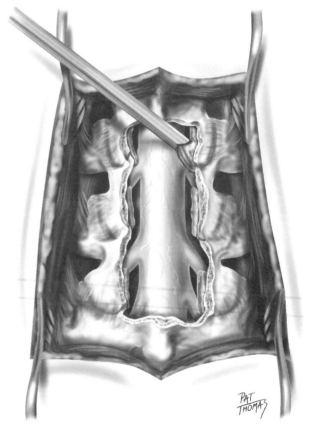

FIGURE 2-1D

Spinous processes and lamina have been removed, thus exposing the thecal sac. At each level, approximately 50% of the facets may be removed without compromising spinal stability.

well as the infolded, frequently calcified ligamentum flavum. In cases of lateral recess or outlet stenosis, the foramina must be meticulously inspected; hemifacetectomy is usually required with lateral recess disease. When more than 50% of the facet is resected bilaterally, consideration should be given to a spinal fusion to prevent the development of iatrogenic spondylolisthesis.

After decompression, the wound is closed in layers over a suction drain. Cellulose or fat is placed over the laminectomy defect. Studies have suggested that the use of a fat graft is more effective and might prevent postoperative adhesions or fibrosis to a greater degree than methylcellulose.

POSTOPERATIVE CARE

The patient is permitted to ambulate as soon as postoperative discomfort permits. Instruction in a flexion program is provided. An orthosis is not necessary in this group.

OUTCOMES

Recent studies have shown that approximately 65% to 70% of patients report significant improvement in ambulatory ability, diminution of pain levels, and overall increase in functional levels after decompressive laminectomy. In patients with residual lower extremity symptoms after laminectomy, residual compression, usually of the lateral recess variety, is the most frequent finding.

COMPLICATIONS

The risk of a dural tear during laminectomy is approximately 4% to 10%. The risk might be higher in patients with dural attenuation as a result of chronic compression from infolded ligamentum flavum or bony elements. Provided the dural tear can be closed with a watertight seal, there is no contraindication to postoperative draining and routine postoperative care after 24 to 48 hours of bed rest.

Delayed complications include development of iatrogenic deformity (spondylolisthesis, kyphosis) or stenosis at an adjacent segment. The risk of development of deformity is related to the amount of decompression; with appropriate sparing of the facets, the risk of delayed spondylolisthesis or kyphosis is less than 2%.

Clinically significant stenosis, resulting in a recurrence of lower extremity symptoms at a segment adjacent to the surgical site, is present in approximately 10% of patients. The results of surgical intervention for the stenosis are markedly inferior to those expected with the primary procedure. The reasons for this are unclear.

3

DEGENERATIVE SPONDYLOLISTHESIS/ STENOSIS

- ## DECOMPRESSIVE LAMINECTOMY – POSTEROLATERAL FUSION

- ## DECOMPRESSIVE LAMINECTOMY – POSTEROLATERAL FUSION

SUMMARY

Degenerative spondylolisthesis is extremely common, with 1 to 3 mm of translation occurring in up to 40% of asymptomatic individuals. In this disease, the spondylolisthesis rarely progresses beyond 25% anterolisthesis because of the intact architecture of the posterior elements. It is thought to be caused by chronic disk degeneration and segmental instability. Facet changes and rotational instability are the rule, with the L_{4-5} level involved most frequently. The vast majority of patients respond to nonoperative care. Decompression with posterolateral fusion is the accepted surgical treatment.

PRESENTATION

Patients will present with back pain from spondylolisthesis and disk degeneration and leg pain due to stenosis. The neurologic presentation can be neuroclaudication

21

or radiculopathy. In central stenosis with resultant neuroclaudication, patients will note activity-related lower extremity pain or heaviness, which will diminish with spinal flexion. Many patients will note increased activity tolerance when ambulating in a flexed position, i.e., walking with a cane, walker, or shopping cart. In cases of lateral recess stenosis with monoradicular symptoms, the nerve root most commonly involved is L_5. These monoradicular symptoms might or might not be related to activity or positional changes, depending on the degree of compression.

NONOPERATIVE CARE

Most patients respond to non-steroidal anti-inflammatory medications, flexion-based physical therapy, and activity modification. There is some evidence that epidural steroid therapy might be beneficial in reducing acute symptoms; however, the long-term benefit of epidural steroid therapy in randomized prospective studies remains unproven.

DIAGNOSTIC STUDIES

Plain films show spondylolisthesis, most typically at L_{4-5}. Flexion and extension x-rays might be beneficial; more than 4 mm of translation between flexion and extension x-rays might indicate significant segmental instability. Whether the patients exhibiting this finding are more likely to fail conservative care and proceed to surgery is unknown.

To assess canal dimensions accurately, MRI is the test of choice. MRI also can provide information regarding underlying marrow changes and the possibility of coexistent neoplasia. In cases where MRI is unavailable or additional bony detail is required, myelography CT is the test of choice. Electrodiagnostic studies (EMG/NCV) have not been found to be useful in the evaluation of this condition.

PROCEDURE

DECOMPRESSIVE LAMINECTOMY – POSTEROLATERAL FUSION (FIG. 3–1)

In patients who have not benefited from appropriate conservative care, decompression with posterolateral fusion in situ is the treatment of choice. The usefulness of this procedure has been convincingly demonstrated in randomized prospective studies; the expectation for improvement in exercise tolerance and pain relief is approximately 85%. Interestingly, this improvement appears to be independent of the status of the arthrodesis because pseudarthrosis has not been associated with a poorer outcome per se.

POSITIONING

The patient is placed prone, in the knee-to-chest position (Fig. 3–1A). Lumbar lordosis is reversed, thus permitting access to the interlaminar spaces.

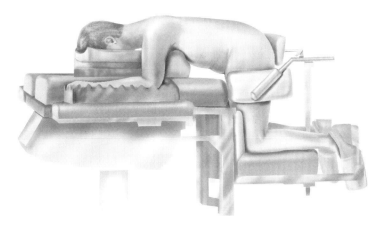

FIGURE 3–1A

**DEGENERATIVE SPONDYLOLISTHESIS AND STENOSIS. DE-
COMPRESSIVE LAMINECTOMY—POSTEROLATERAL FUSION.**
The patient is positioned prone in a standard knee-to-chest
configuration, with the abdomen hanging free.

TECHNIQUE

An incision is made in the midline, most frequently over L_{4-5}, and extending the
length of the area to be decompressed (Fig. 3–1B). Dissection is carried down to
the fascia and self-retaining retractors are inserted. The fascia is incised on either
side of the midline and reflected laterally to the facets. In the levels that are to be
fused, a far lateral dissection then follows, with stripping of the posterior spinous
musculature, including the multifidus, from the appropriate transverse processes.

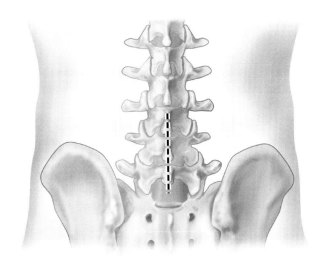

FIGURE 3–1B

A skin incision is made from L_{3-4} to $L_5–S_1$.

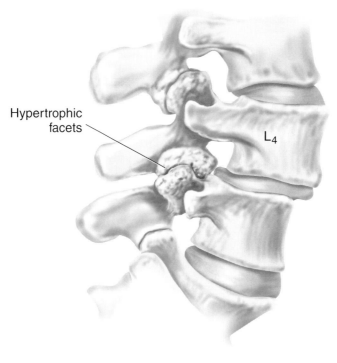

Hypertrophic
facets

L₄

FIGURE 3-1C

Degenerative spondylolisthesis is rarely greater than 25% translation of L₄ on L₅. Note degenerative changes in the facets, resulting in foraminal outlet stenosis, and the intact pars.

On the lateral projection, hypertrophic defects are visible at the level of the spondylolysis (Fig. 3–1C).

Supraspinous and intraspinous ligaments are then removed with the spinous processes of the levels undergoing decompression. After thinning of the lamina as necessary, a laminectomy is performed with a high-speed burr and completed with a Kerrison rongeur (Fig. 3–1D). Complete facetectomy may be performed at the level at which arthrodesis is undertaken; care must be taken at adjacent levels. If more than 50% of the involved facets are resected for adequate neural decompression, then posterolateral fusion is indicated (Fig. 3–1E). A thorough decompression of the subarticular and central components is important. The ligamentum flavum may be infolded and should be resected meticulously.

After decompression, iliac crest autograft is harvested through the same incision or a separate incision in the standard manner. Care should be taken to remain within a 6-cm radius of the posterosuperior iliac spine because more exuberant graft harvesting might lead to an unacceptably high incidence of persistent pain, formation of cluneal neuromata, or dissatisfaction with wound cosmesis.

The wound is then closed over suction drainage in appropriate layers.

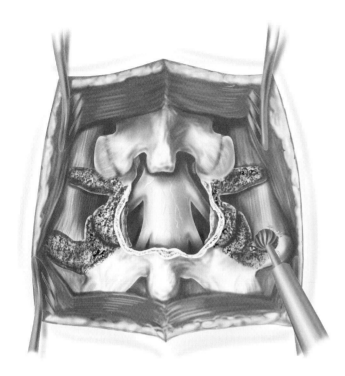

FIGURE 3-1D

The spine is exposed to the tips of the transverse processes. Complete laminectomy at L_4 and partial laminectomy of L_5 were performed. Facetectomy can be partial, as illustrated here, or complete, depending on the extent of decompression required. The L_4 and L_5 transverse processes and the lateral aspect of the zygapophyseal joint at L_{4-5} were decorticated with a high-speed burr. The L_{3-4} facet was not violated.

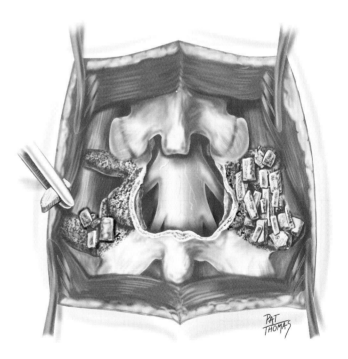

FIGURE 3-1E

Graft is placed into both gutters.

POSTOPERATIVE CARE

The patient is encouraged to ambulate as soon as possible after surgery. The use of a postoperative orthosis is a matter of individual preference. There has been no reported augmentation of arthrodesis rates related to the use of an orthosis. If an orthosis is selected, it should be recalled that, for the lumbosacral junction to be immobilized effectively, a thigh cuff or other leg extension is needed.

OUTCOMES

Approximately 85% of patients have reported improved exercise tolerance and diminished pain as a result of this procedure. The addition of arthrodesis to decompression to treat the spondylolisthesis diminishes the likelihood of progressive listhesis and is associated with improved outcomes.

COMPLICATIONS

As with any spinal procedure, there is a risk of dural injury intraoperatively resulting in dural lacerations (0.5%). Tears should be repaired in a watertight manner if possible; if this is accomplished, then no significant clinical sequelae are expected. In cases of persistent postoperative headache or drainage of cerebrospinal fluid through the operative wound (dural cutaneous fistula), closed subarachnoid drainage has been shown to be successful in a high percentage of cases. Most instances of dural cutaneous fistula will seal after 3 to 4 days of closed subarachnoid drainage, thus obviating the need for additional surgery.

4

DEGENERATIVE SCOLIOSIS/STENOSIS

- ## DECOMPRESSIVE LAMINECTOMY/ INSTRUMENTED FUSION

- ## DECOMPRESSIVE LAMINECTOMY/ INSTRUMENTED FUSION

SUMMARY

Scoliosis is a disease with two age peaks epidemiologically. The first is in adolescence and the second occurs in the sixth or seventh decade of life, presumably on the basis of asymmetric degenerative change. That change is characterized by a lateral listhesis as opposed to rotational deformity, seldom exceeds 45 degrees, and is invariably of the lumbar variety. Of course, adolescent idiopathic curves also can persist into adulthood. Although the curves themselves are no more likely to be more symptomatic from degenerative change than other age-matched controls, this condition is frequently associated with lumbar spinal stenosis. The principles of treatment for this type of stenosis are similar to those for stenosis with a straight spine. However, the presence of deformity clearly changes surgical management.

PRESENTATION

The patient with degenerative scoliosis and stenosis frequently presents with non-specific complaints, as is the case in the patient with lumbar spinal stenosis. Complaints include backache, unilateral or bilateral leg pain, or activity-related lower extremity pain (neural claudication.) As a rule, the neurologic examination is normal. Root tension signs are often absent. Occasionally, if lateral recess stenosis is present, the patient might exhibit referred radicular pain in an extremity, a finding associated with side-gliding toward that extremity. It can be exacerbated by extension of the spine if there also is significant lateral recess encroachment. Signs of a classic scoliotic deformity (rib prominence) are usually not present in cases of lumbar scoliosis and stenosis because the thoracic spine is seldom involved and the rotational component of the deformity is not as pronounced as in adolescent scoliosis. Diminished lumbar lordosis, the so-called flat back, may be present.

NONOPERATIVE CARE

Nonoperative care consists of nonsteroidal anti-inflammatory medications and physical therapy. The role of epidural steroids remains unproven but the drugs might be useful in diminishing initial symptoms so as to make long-term maintenance with nonsteroidal anti-inflammatory medications or physical therapy more promising. Although certain therapy regimens involving flexion and distraction of the spine have proven promising in the treatment of this condition, convincing data on these protocols are notably absent. The use of supportive corsets and braces has been shown to be of no value whatsoever.

DIAGNOSTIC STUDIES

Plain films show lumbar scoliosis. MRI frequently is not useful in determining the extent and degree of compression caused by the deformity. In that instance, CT myelography is invaluable in providing information concerning canal dimensions, foraminal dimensions, and the relation of the cauda equina to the canal.

PROCEDURE

DECOMPRESSIVE LAMINECTOMY/INSTRUMENTED FUSION (FIG. 4–1):

The procedure of choice is decompression in concert with spinal fusion and, if possible, correction of the deformity.

POSITIONING

The patient is placed on a roll or in a modified knee-to-chest position to reconstitute lumbar contours (Fig. 4–1A), which may not be possible because of the loss of lordosis associated with scoliosis and the segmental changes preventing positional correction of the deformity. After all extremities are padded, the posterior lumbar spine is prepared and draped into the sterile field. An incision is made in the midline (Fig. 4–1B). A posterior approach to expose the degenerative curve then follows (Fig. 4–1C).

Laminectomy is performed in a standard manner with a high-speed burr, Kerrison rongeurs, curettes, and Leksell and Kerrison rongeurs. A wide decompression is required, with particular attention to foraminal decompression on the concavity of the curve. Wide facetectomy is the rule.

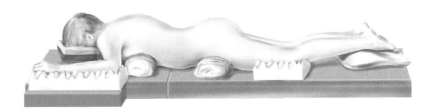

FIGURE 4–1A

**DEGENERATIVE SCOLIOSIS AND STENOSIS. DECOMPRES-
SIVE LAMINECTOMY.** The patient is positioned on rolls under
the sternum and pelvis, with the abdomen hanging free.
Extremities are padded.

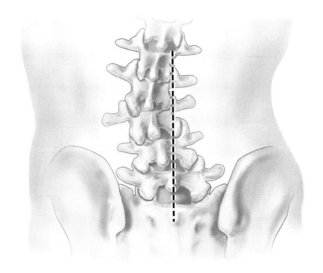

FIGURE 4–1B

A midline skin incision is made from L_1 to the sacrum.

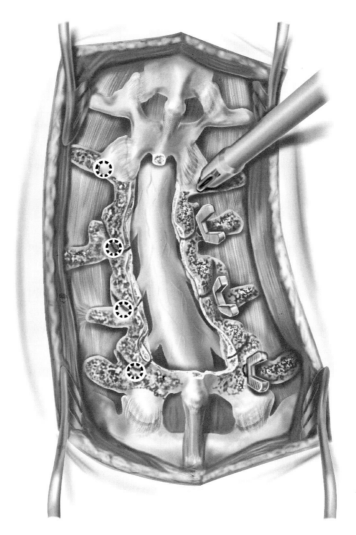

FIGURE 4-1C

The spine is exposed to the tips of the transverse processes bilaterally. Complete laminectomy is performed as necessary. In this instance, care must be taken not to damage the L_{1-2} or L_5–S_1 facets.

At the conclusion of the procedure, the exiting nerve roots should be clearly visualized at all levels, with removal of all osteophytic prominences and infolded ligamentum flavum.

The transverse processes are then exposed and decorticated with a high-speed burr or osteotome. Local autograft and autograft harvested from the iliac crest are then placed into the gutters. Particular attention should be given to decorticating the lateral aspect of the remnants of the zygapophyseal joints because these might represent up to 20% of the surface area available for grafting. Segmental instrumenta-

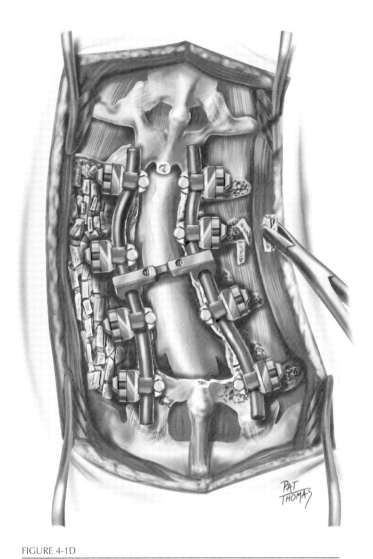

FIGURE 4-1D

Segmental instrumentation is placed, followed by construct assembly and posterolateral grafting.

tion, usually in the form of interpedicular screws, is then placed (Fig. 4–1D). Gel foam, fat grafts, or newer substitutes to prevent dural adhesions are then placed over the laminectomy; the wound is then closed in layers over suction drains.

POSTOPERATIVE CARE

The value of bracing is not clear in cases where instrumentation has been used. The patient should be mobilized as quickly as possible and encouraged to ambulate with whatever aids are necessary. An inpatient rehabilitation program for these patients might be desirable but not beneficial in terms of eventual outcome. Drains are removed by the second postoperative day and intravenous sedation in the form of patient-controlled analgesia is converted to oral medication.

OUTCOMES

Approximately 70% of patients treated surgically for degenerative scoliosis have reported satisfactory pain relief and increased ambulatory ability.

COMPLICATIONS

Complications are hardware failure and loosening, hardware breakage, pseudarthrosis and collapse, and junctional stenosis. In most constrained hardware systems, hardware failure per se should not be a significant factor (incidence, 0.5%). Junctional stenosis, i.e., stenosis at the rostral or caudal edge of the decompression, is becoming a more frequently recognized problem. Certain investigators have reported bony overgrowth in up to 88% of these cases, but the true frequency of symptomatic stenosis is not known.

5

SPONDYLOLISTHESIS

- GILL LAMINECTOMY AND FUSION WITH INSTRUMENTATION
- LUMBOSACRAL FUSION IN SITU

- GILL LAMINECTOMY AND FUSION WITH INSTRUMENTATION

- LUMBOSACRAL FUSION IN SITU

SUMMARY

Spondylolisthesis is a sagittal deformity characterized by the anterior displacement of one vertebra with respect to its neighbor. The Meyerding classification (grades I through V) is widely accepted. The degree of translation of one vertebra with regard to the other is graded as a percentage of slip based on the superior end-plate of the caudal vertebra: grade I, slips up to 25%; grade II, 25% to 50%; grade III, 50% to 75%; grade IV, 75% to 100%; and grade V, or spondyloptosis, which implies complete translocation of the vertebra from its adjacent caudal segment.

PRESENTATION

Congenital spondylolisthesis is associated with dysplasia of the articular processes and elongation or discontinuity of the pars articularis. If the pars is intact, these slips are usually no greater than grade II. The incidence of lytic spondylolisthesis (pars not intact) is approximately 1% at the age of 18 years. Many patients with lytic spondylolisthesis also have associated abnormalities of posterior elements at the level of the spondylolisthesis involving the superior articular process. These particular types of spondylolisthesis occur at L_5–S_1. Degenerative spondylolisthesis occurs at L_4–5 and is associated with stenosis, as noted in Chap. 4. Posttraumatic spondylolisthesis involves a fracture of the pars interarticularis. Such a fracture is usually apparent in an adoles-

33

cent who has sustained a traumatic episode and has an unusually high prevalence in female gymnasts. Pathologic spondylolisthesis and post-surgical spondylolisthesis obviously are recognized in the appropriate setting.

In general, patients with a grade I or higher slip have higher incidences of back pain than the general population. In adolescence, the patient presenting with a grade II slip, or a slip angle larger than 40 degrees, is a candidate for arthrodesis. If neither a high-grade nor progressive slip is present, the pain is not intolerable, and there is no neurologic deficit, conservative care is indicated initially.

NONOPERATIVE CARE

In the pediatric population, a brief period of rest, orthosis wear, or activity modification might resolve symptoms and can take up to 3 months. This rest period is followed by physical therapy in the form of flexion exercises and trunk strengthening. The slip should be monitored periodically with x-rays.

In adults, once neoplasm or progressive deformity is ruled out, anti-inflammatory medications, hamstring stretching, and appropriate physical therapy are the treatments of choice. In the adult, there has been no demonstrated value of orthotic wear.

DIAGNOSTIC STUDIES

Plain x-rays are diagnostic. If additional information is desired, MRI is the method of choice to image canal dimensions more completely and assess the state of disk hydration in the adult patient. For superior neuroforaminal detail, particularly of the lumbosacral segment, CT myelography is the procedure of choice. With a high slip angle and anterior translation, the pedicle of L_5 frequently compresses the exiting L_5 root against the lateral sacral promontory. The L_5 root also can be tented posteriorly. The remaining sacral nerve roots are subject to traction.

PROCEDURES

GILL LAMINECTOMY AND FUSION WITH INSTRUMENTATION (FIG. 5–1)

POSITIONING

The patient is placed in a knee-to-chest or 90–90 position with as much flexion as is tolerated to open the canal and aid in partial reduction of the deformity (Fig. 5–1A). A midline incision is then made and the autogenous iliac crest bone is harvested through a separate incision or a suprafascial dissection from the midline (Fig. 5–1B). In the lateral projection, the pars defect at L_5 is clearly seen (Fig. 5–1C).

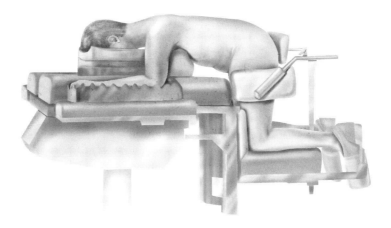

FIGURE 5–1A

SPONDYLOLISTHESIS—GILL LAMINECTOMY AND FUSION WITH INSTRUMENTATION. The patient is positioned prone in a standard knee-to-chest configuration, with the abdomen hanging free.

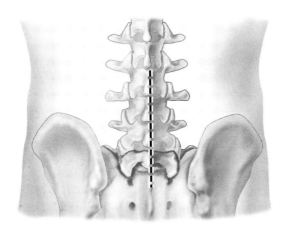

FIGURE 5–1B

A midline skin incision is made from L_3 to the sacrum.

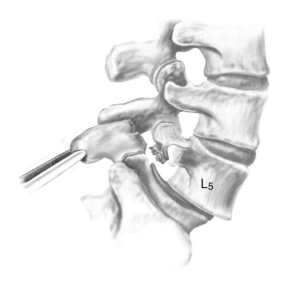

FIGURE 5-1C

In lumbosacral isthmic spondylolisthesis, L_5 is displaced anteriorly and inferiorly. This results in L_5–S_1 foraminal stenosis, with the L_5 transverse processes situated directly anterior to the sacral alae. Due to the pars defect, the L_5 lamina (Gill fragment) is hypermobile.

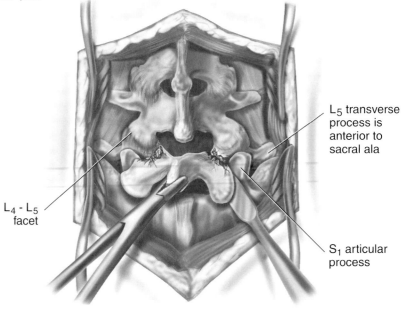

FIGURE 5-1D

A wide exposure is necessary to visualize the transverse processes of L_5 and the sacral alae. The Gill fragment is removed by sharp and blunt dissection. Residual ligamentum flavum and osseous material are resected with a Kerrison rongeur after Gill laminectomy.

TECHNIQUE

In cases of significant neural compression, laminectomy is indicated. The incision is made in the midline and carried down to the posterior elements. A lateral spinal dissection follows, with reflection of the muscle out to the facet. A far lateral dissection is the next step, with exposure of the transverse processes of L_5 and the sacral ala (Fig. 5–1D). The deep layer of the multifidus muscle is sacrificed. In general, in cases where the slip exceeds 50%, arthrodesis may be carried rostrally to L_4 and exposure should involve that level as well.

In the discontinuous congenital and lytic varieties of spondylolisthesis, the posterior arch of L_5 (Gill fragment) is immediately evident; this will be loose and easily mobilized. The arch is removed in the standard manner after dissecting the ligamentum flavum free and establishing a plane in the canal (Fig. 5–1E). Upon removal, the loose cartilaginous anlage may be evident as remnants of the pars. Decompression is then performed to expose the L_5 and S_1 nerve roots. Typically, the pedicles of L_5 and the transverse processes are extremely anterior to the sacrum. A complete facetectomy with foraminotomy at L_5–S_1 is required. If necessary, L_4 also is decompressed.

Fusion is then performed with instrumentation (Fig. 5–1F). Interpedicular instrumentation is the fixation of choice for fusing L_5–S_1, L_4–$_5$, or L_4–$_5$ and L_5–S_1. The bone graft is placed in the decorticated gutters, taking care to decorticate any remnants of the lateral zygapophyseal processes. Instrumentation is then placed. The laminectomy defect is covered with cellulose or fat graft and the wound is closed in layers over a suction drain.

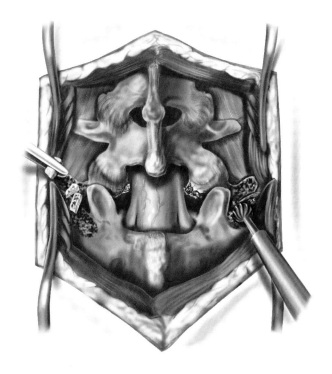

FIGURE 5-1E

The transverse processes of L_5 and the sacral alae are decorticated. Bone graft is placed bilaterally.

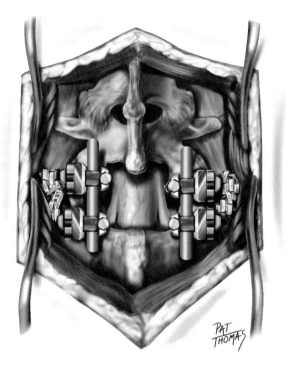

FIGURE 5-1F

Interpedicular fixation is placed at L$_5$–S$_1$. Because of the anterior translation of L$_5$, the L$_5$–S$_1$ interpedicular distance is shortened in the coronal plane; thus, screws placed in those segments might touch.

In cases where there is no significant neural compression, a lumbosacral fusion in situ may be performed. The procedure can be performed through a midline approach or two parallel paraspinous approaches. In cases of spondylolisthesis of grade II or greater, consideration should be given to extending the fusion to L$_4$; for lower grade slips, lumbosacral fusion (L$_5$–S$_1$) will suffice.

In the midline approach, after appropriate positioning, the patient is prepared and draped into a sterile field and an incision is made. A lateral spinal dissection then follows in a manner analogous to that described above. Once the transverse processes are exposed, the bone graft is placed. During the approach, care must be taken not to disrupt the supraspinous and intraspinous ligaments at L$_{4-5}$ or S$_1$. The wound is then closed in layers over a suction drain.

In the paraspinous approach, two parallel incisions are made adjacent to the midline, right and left approximately 4 to 5 cm from the midline, or over the level of the facets. The muscle layers are split and self-retaining retractors are inserted. Dissection is carried down to the lateral margins of the facet and out onto the transverse processes from which the deep layer of the multifidus is reflected. Bone graft, harvested from a separate fascial incision, is then placed on the decorticated spinous processes and the wounds are closed in layers over suction drains.

POSTOPERATIVE CARE

The benefit of postoperative orthotic wear is unclear in the cases of Gill laminec-tomy, fusion, and fusion in situ. Many studies, particularly in adolescents, have sug-gested a higher rate of arthrodesis, with fusion in situ if an orthosis is used. If an orthosis is to be used, it must include a thigh cuff to provide immobilization across the lumbosacral junction. In younger children, a pantaloon spica may be a viable alternative.

OUTCOMES

In adolescents, the fusion rate approximates 95%. That rate also closely approxi-mates the rate of clinical success in terms of pain relief. Postoperatively, it is imper-ative that the patient continues with a therapy program emphasizing hamstring stretching.

In the adult, the results regarding pain relief are less optimistic, although a suc-cessful outcome regarding back and leg pain is attained in more than 80% of indi-viduals. The use of internal fixation in securing arthrodesis can result in a union rate of 80% to 85%.

COMPLICATIONS

In instrumented fusions, complications are hardware failure, pseudarthrosis, and fail-ure to obtain pain relief. In those adolescents with large slip angles that are not reduced, a compensatory hyperlordosis might develop. The hyperlordosis might result in hamstring tightness and gait abnormalities. In patients with slip angles larger than 40 degrees, preoperative traction to reduce the slip angle may be indicated.

Although some investigators advocate reduction of spondylolisthesis in the sagit-tal plane, the usefulness of this as compared with fusion in situ with reduction of the slip angle has not been convincingly demonstrated.

LUMBOSACRAL FUSION IN SITU (FIG. 5–2)

POSITIONING

The patient is placed in a knee-to-chest or 90–90 position with as much flexion as is tolerated to open the canal and aid in partial reduction of the deformity (Fig. 5–2A).

TECHNIQUE

The classic surgical approach for stabilization of lumbosacral spondylolisthesis is posterolateral fusion in situ (Wiltse). With this approach, the midline elements including the Gill fragment and supraspinous and intraspinous ligaments are not vio-lated. Posterolateral bone grafting between the transverse processes of L_5 and the sacral alae in cases of low grade slips (grade II or less) is the key to the operation.

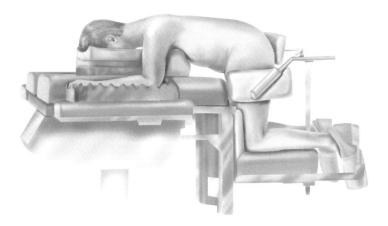

FIGURE 5–2A

SPONDYLOLISTHESIS LUMBOSACRAL FUSION IN SITU. The patient is positioned prone in a standard knee-to-chest configuration, with the abdomen hanging free.

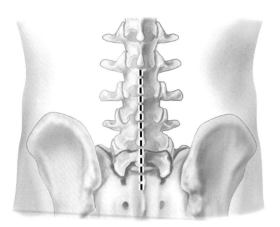

FIGURE 5–2B

A midline skin incision is made from L₃ to the sacrum. Subcutaneous tissue is retracted to expose fascia. Fascial incisions are made bilaterally, two to three fingerbreadths lateral to the facets.

With higher grade slips (grades II through V), posterolateral fusion from L₄ to the sacrum is indicated.

After positioning, the incision spanning the defect and the lumbosacral junction is made (Figs. 5–2B and C). Bilateral incisions can be made approximately two to three fingerbreadths from the midline, or a single midline incision can be made. In the case of a single midline skin incision, dissection is carried down to the fascia and self-retaining retractors are inserted. The fascia is then split longitudinally two to three fingerbreadths from the midline bilaterally and dissection is carried anteriorly. In cases of bilateral skin incisions, the dissection is carried straight through the fascia anteriorly, lateral to the facets, thereby exposing the transverse processes (Fig. 5–2D). The muscle dissection is performed bluntly with Cobb elevators and hand-held retractors as indicated. Unipolar electrocautery is used for hemostasis

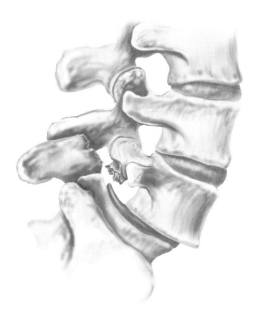

FIGURE 5-2C

In lumbosacral isthmic spondylolisthesis, L_5 is displaced anteriorly and inferiorly, resulting in L_5–S_1 foraminal stenosis, with the L_5 transverse processes situated directly anterior to the sacral alae. Due to the pars defect, the L_5 lamina (Gill fragment) is hypermobile.

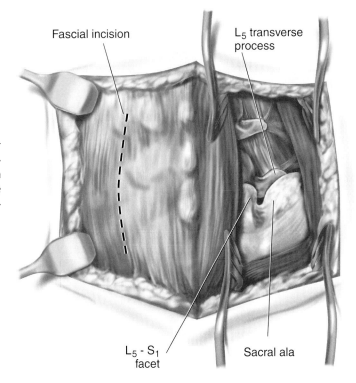

FIGURE 5-2D

The transverse processes of L_4 and L_5 are exposed with the sacral alae. Midline musculature is not disturbed. The dotted line on the left indicates the location of the fascial incision. On the right, the fascia is split, with exposure of the transverse processes and alae.

and to dissect the deep layer of the multifidus muscle off of the transverse processes. The iliolumbar ligament frequently must be split as well to expose the sacral alae.

Iliac crest bone graft is then harvested through a transverse or curvilinear incision beginning inferiorly at the level of the posterosuperior iliac spine. Self-retaining retractors are inserted and hemostasis is obtained with electrocautery. The gluteal fascia is thus exposed and incised in line with the iliac crest. With Cobb elevators and electrocautery, the gluteus medius is reflected laterally. Directly anterior and slightly inferior to the superior iliac spine, the gluteal notch can be palpated. Because of the risk of neurovascular injury, this structure should be avoided; this is easily accomplished by keeping the graft harvest rostral to the notch. Osteotomes and gouges are then used to harvest multiple cortical and cancellous strips in the usual manner.

The harvested graft is then divided into equal halves and, after decortication of the posterolateral troughs, the graft is placed through the lateral incisions (Fig. 5–2E). Care should be taken to decorticate the lateral aspect of the zygapophyseal joints as well as the transverse process and alae.

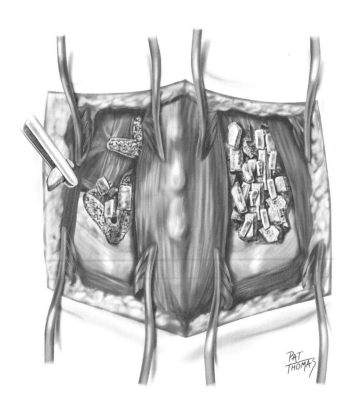

FIGURE 5-2E

The transverse processes and the lateral zygapophyseal joints at L$_{4-5}$ and L$_5$–S$_1$ are decorticated. Bone graft is placed.

The retractors are removed and the wound is closed in layers. Because the canal has not been violated, routine closed suction drainage is not indicated. This may, of course, be performed depending on the specifics of the case and the individual surgeon's preference.

POSTOPERATIVE CARE

The benefit of postoperative orthotic wear is unclear in the cases of Gill laminectomy, fusion, and fusion in situ. Many studies, particularly in adolescents, have suggested a higher rate of arthrodesis with fusion in situ if an orthosis is used. If an orthosis is to be used, it must include a thigh cuff to provide immobilization across the lumbosacral junction. In younger children, a pantaloon spica may be a viable alternative.

OUTCOMES

In adolescents, the fusion rate approximates 95%. That rate also closely approximates the rate of clinical success in terms of pain relief. Postoperatively, it is imperative that the patient continues with a therapy program emphasizing hamstring stretching.

In the adult, the results regarding pain relief are less optimistic, although a successful outcome regarding back and leg pain is attained in more than 80% of individuals. The use of internal fixation in securing arthrodesis can result in a union rate of 80% to 85%.

COMPLICATIONS

In those adolescents with a large slip angle that is not reduced, compensatory hyperlordosis can develop and result in hamstring tightness and gait abnormalities. In patients with slip angle larger than 40 degrees, preoperative traction to reduce the slip angle may be indicated.

6

LOW BACK PAIN

- POSTERIOR INTERBODY FUSION WITH BONE GRAFTS
- ANTERIOR LUMBAR INTERBODY FUSION WITH CAGES
- POSTEROLATERAL FUSION WITH INSTRUMENTATION

- POSTERIOR INTERBODY FUSION WITH BONE GRAFTS

- ANTERIOR LUMBAR INTERBODY FUSION WITH CAGES

- POSTEROLATERAL FUSION WITH INSTRUMENTATION

SUMMARY

Low back pain is ubiquitous. Eighty percent of individuals suffer an episode lasting from 1 to 3 days. Prognosis was thought to be excellent, with recovery from the initial episode as the rule. However, more recent data have suggested that there is a high rate of recurrence of low back pain and that the natural history may be far from benign. Unfortunately, few studies to date have been able to demonstrate optimal nonoperative care.

PRESENTATION

Patients will present with low back pain and nonradicular lower extremity pain. The pain typically will be at the belt line, extending rostrally not beyond the thoracolumbar junction. Distal radiation, as a rule, does not extend beyond the knee.

A thorough history should be taken. In general, pain related to anterior structures (e.g., intervertebral disk) is reduced in extension. Patients thus will report improvement with standing or recumbency. Intradiskal pressure has been shown to be higher while sitting than while standing; as a result, these patients report more pain while sitting or when exposed to vibratory stimuli in a sitting position (e.g., driving). Patients with posterior mechanical pain (facet or spondylolysis) typically have a flexion preference and are improved with sitting. Hamstring tightness may or may not be noted with this group. Neurological examination is, as a rule, normal.

NONOPERATIVE CARE

A short course of nonsteroidal drugs and a brief period of bed rest, not to exceed 72 hours, have been shown to be of benefit in shortening symptomatic intervals. Although many varieties of conservative care including manipulation and physical therapy have been advocated, none has been shown to be superior to the other or from simple observation in randomized controlled trials.

DIAGNOSTIC STUDIES

Plain films may show disk space narrowing, but this is extraordinarily non-specific. The test of choice is MRI. In low back pain without stenosis or deformity, changes on MRI will be limited to disk desiccation on T2-weighted images and disk space narrowing. The MRI is quite sensitive but non-specific. In one study of asymptomatic individuals, only 36% had normal disks at all levels.

If a diskogenic etiology is suspected, the next line of investigation is provocative diskography. In this procedure, whereby x-ray contrast (or saline in a contrast-allergic individual) is injected in the intervertebral disk space, information of two sorts is obtained. The first is morphologic, characterizing degenerative changes. The second, more valuable category is clinical. If, upon injection, concordant pain is reproduced, then the test is considered to be positive. A recent study has shown that, in the correct hands, sensitivity and specificity rates with diskography are quite high. The test, however, remains controversial due to problems with application and the essentially subjective nature of the test (concordant pain reproduction).

In patients with suspected symptomatic facets, a facet block may be performed. However, those blocks have been shown to be predominantly therapeutic. Because each facet receives significant cross-innervation from adjacent levels, specificity of this technique is limited, and certainly, without a defect in the pars or spondylolisthesis, no surgical intervention can be recommended on the basis of facet studies alone.

Selective nerve root sheath injections ("nerve root blocks") have been shown to be neither sensitive nor specific.

PROCEDURES

POSTERIOR INTERBODY FUSION WITH BONE GRAFTS (FIG. 6–1)

POSITIONING

For the posterior procedures, the patient is placed prone, with the knees slightly flexed or in a knee-to-chest position (Fig. 6–1A). Either position will tend to open the intervertebral spaces but also result in a loss of lordosis. To circumvent this difficulty, the use of a prone positioning table has been advocated, but this significantly impedes access to the disk space.

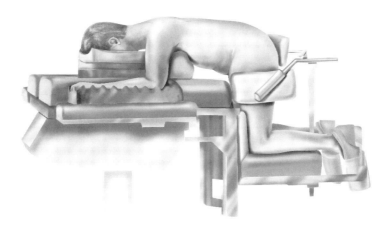

FIGURE 6–1A

POSTERIOR INTERBODY FUSION WITH BONE GRAFT. The patient is positioned prone in a standard knee-to-chest configuration, with the abdomen hanging free.

TECHNIQUE

A midline incision is made and a posterior spinal dissection follows in the usual manner, with stripping of the spinous musculature to the facets (Fig. 6–1B). The transverse processes need not be exposed in this procedure because these will not be grafted. Self-retaining retractors are then inserted.

The correct level is identified with static films or fluoroscopy. A laminotomy is then performed by removal of intraspinous and supraspinous ligaments and laminectomy and hemifacetectomy with a high-speed burr and appropriate Kerrison

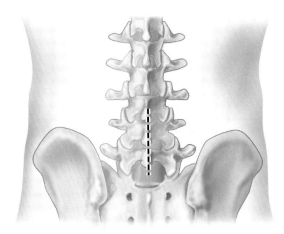

FIGURE 6–1B

For an L$_{4-5}$ posterior interbody fusion, a midline skin incision is made from L$_3$ to L$_5$.

rongeurs. Bipolar electrocautery is used to control bleeding in the canal and the thecal sac is then gently retracted bilaterally in a sequential manner. A thorough diskectomy is performed right and left, with curetting of the cartilaginous end-plates (Fig. 6–1C). Care should be taken not to perforate the end-plates.

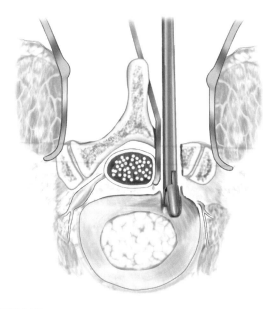

FIGURE 6-1C

For proper insertion of an interbody graft, a large laminotomy is performed, which permits sequential retraction of the neural elements to the midline bilaterally. Dorsal exposure need not be carried lateral to the facets.

Tricortical grafts are then harvested from the iliac crest by a separate incision or a suprafascial dissection from the main wound. It is imperative that the iliac crest be exposed in such a manner that a tricortical graft of the appropriate dimensions can be taken. Additional cortical and cancellous bone is removed.

Attention is then returned to the surgical field. Taking care to protect the nerve roots, a small box osteotome is used to cut rectangular troughs on the right and left sides of the disk space to a depth not exceeding 2 mm (Fig. 6–1D). The tricortical grafts are then fashioned to accommodate these troughs and impacted (Fig. 6–1E). Additional cortical cancellous graft is packed around them.

A final check is made for bleeding and the laminotomy is then covered with a fat graft or cellulose. A suction drain is placed in the depths of the wound and the muscles are returned to the midline and closed. The remainder of the wound is closed in layers.

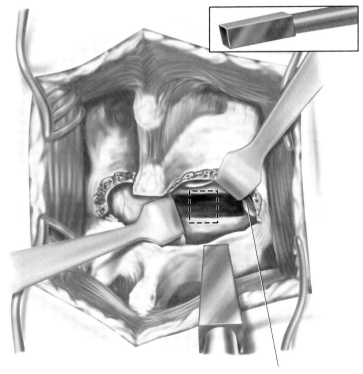

L₄ nerve root

FIGURE 6-1D

The L$_{4-5}$ segment is exposed. A generous laminotomy is performed, with partial excision of the L$_4$ spinous process. The thecal sac is mobilized and retracted toward the midline. An annular window is removed and the disk space is prepared with a box osteotome (insert).

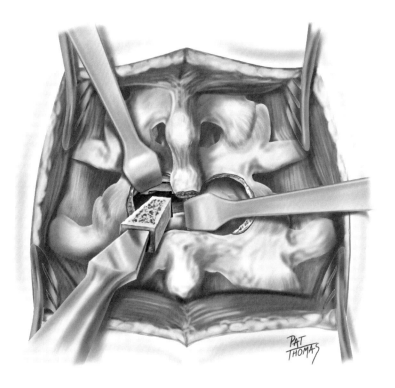

FIGURE 6-1E

Care must be taken to protect the exiting nerve roots at the rostral and caudal levels (in this instance, L_4 and L_5). The L_4 root is taken laterally and the L_5 root is taken medially. A tricortical graft is inserted. The procedure is then repeated on the opposite side.

ANTERIOR LUMBAR INTERBODY FUSION WITH CAGES (FIG. 6–2)

When performing surgery anteriorly, stability is obtained with interbody instrumentation without disturbing the structural integrity of the posterior column or the neural elements. In a sense, this is a more physiologic approach and virtually eliminates the risk of postoperative epidural fibrosis. Anterior interbody fusion with threaded cages can be performed from a laparoscopic approach at L_5–S_1 or an open extra- or transperitoneal approach.

POSITIONING

In all instances, the patient is positioned supine with the knees extended and the operating table in a jack-knifed position (Fig. 6–2A). This accentuates the lordosis and affords access to the interbody spaces.

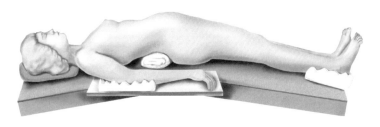

FIGURE 6–2A

ANTERIOR INTERBODY FUSION WITH CAGES. The patient is positioned supine with the spine extended.

TECHNIQUE

For laparoscopic anterior interbody fusion, the assistance of a trained laparoscopic surgeon is required. Two portals are created in the abdomen, one at the umbilicus and the other superior to the pubis in line with the L_5–S_1 disk space. Currently, the L_5–S_1 disk space is the only one routinely accessible with the laparoscope due to the more proximal position of the bifurcation of the great vessels. With CO_2 insufflated into the abdomen and the patient in a reverse Trendelenburg position, the laparoscopic surgeon will mobilize the colon, divide the anterior sacral artery, and mobilize and retract the great vessels, thus exposing the L_5–S_1 disk space. Bone graft is harvested through a small incision lateral to the anterosuperior iliac spine and used to pack the interbody cages. Cage insertion will be described shortly during the open approach. All laparoscopic wounds are closed in layers with appropriate sutures.

The direct anterior approach is most frequently performed through a paramedian incision to preserve the rectus muscle (Fig. 6–2B). The transperitoneal exposure

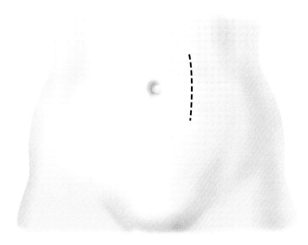

FIGURE 6–2B

The skin incision is made three fingerbreadths lateral to the umbilicus, extending proximally and distally, for approximately 4 cm.

is more extensive. The peritoneum is divided in the midline and the abdominal contents are mobilized and protected. The superior hypogastric plexus provides sympathetic innervation of the urogenital system. These nerves extend across the left iliac vessels, the fifth lumbar body, and the lumbosacral junction. These might be injured during the approach. When the posterior peritoneum is incised longitudinally, the iliacs are identified and mobilized and the right ureter should be identified. After blunt tissue mobilization, the appropriate disk spaces are visualized.

Alternatively, the spine can be approached extraperitoneally. This is most commonly done by a left-sided approach posteriorly along the renal fascia, behind the ureter. This prevents direct injury to the hypogastric plexus. The abdominal contents are reflected en bloc and the spine is visualized.

Cage insertion is performed in a similar manner regardless of exposure. The initial step involves incision of the disk space, followed by appropriate distraction and insertion of a sleeve, to permit passage of reamers and protect abdominal contents (Fig. 6–2C). The midline should be localized with x-ray or fluoroscopy to facilitate symmetric insertion of cages. Each tract is then appropriately reamed, cleaned with a Kerrison rongeur, tapped, and filled with the cages packed with graft (Fig. 6–2D). X-ray or fluoroscopic verification of cage size is imperative to prevent encroachment into the spinal canal.

The wounds are then closed in a standard manner.

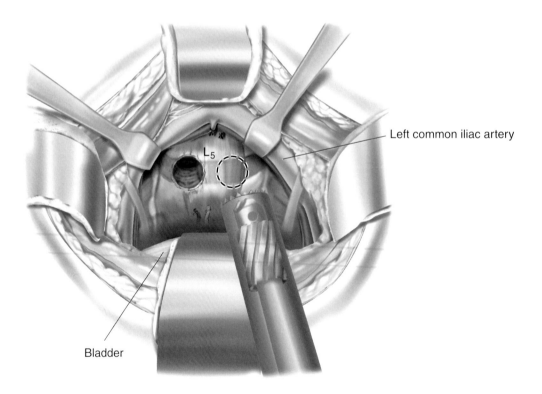

FIGURE 6-2C

In the transperitoneal approach, the peritoneum is divided and the great vessels are retracted laterally. The midline is located and verified with x-ray or fluoroscopic guidance. The interspace is prepared.

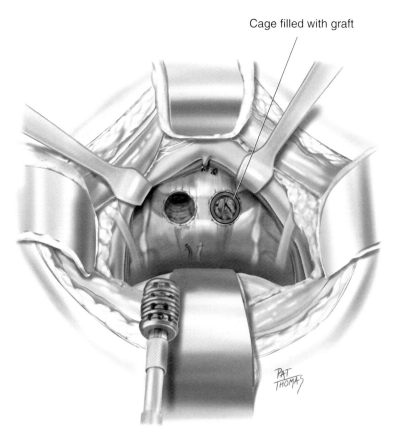

Cage filled with graft

FIGURE 6-2D

The annulus is incised bilaterally and partial diskectomy, reaming, and tapping are performed. A threaded cage is packed with bone graft and inserted. The procedure is then repeated on the opposite side.

POSTEROLATERAL FUSION WITH INSTRUMENTATION (FIG. 6–3)

POSITIONING

The patient is placed prone and with the knees slightly flexed or in a knee-to-chest position (Fig. 6–3A).

TECHNIQUE

A standard midline posterior incision is made and the spine exposed and decorticated (Figs. 6–3B and C).

Interpedicular instrumentation can be placed in one of several ways. If the procedure is to be done in a closed manner (i.e., without opening the spinal

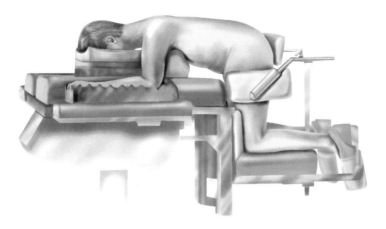

FIGURE 6–3A

POSTEROLATERAL FUSION WITH INSTRUMENTATION. The patient is positioned prone, with the knees slightly flexed or in a knee-to-chest position.

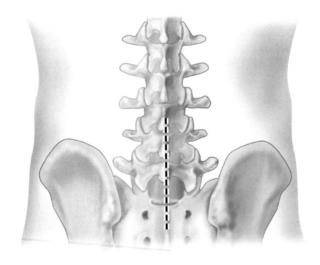

FIGURE 6–3B

A midline skin incision is made from L$_3$ to the sacrum.

canal), a point just lateral to the facets and in the midpoint of the transverse processes is selected. The cortex is broached with a high-speed burr and a probe is inserted into the pedicle (Fig. 6–3D). This is done under fluoroscopic guidance. Once the correct screw length has been selected, the hole is tapped and the screw is inserted.

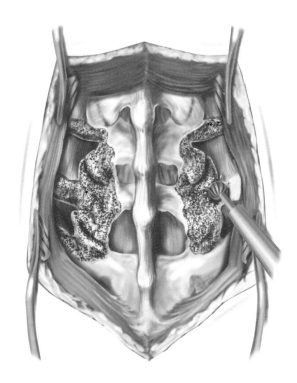

FIGURE 6-3C

Posterior exposure is performed laterally to the tips of the transverse processes. These are decorticated with the corresponding aspects of the lateral zygapophyseal joints and sacral alae. The L$_{3-4}$ facets should not be violated.

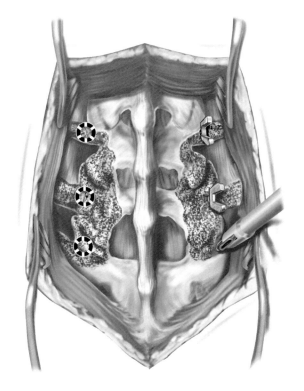

FIGURE 6-3D

Screw insertion can be performed in an open or closed manner. The appropriate target for screw insertion is determined by the intersection of a line bisecting the transverse process with the lateral edge of the facet at that level.

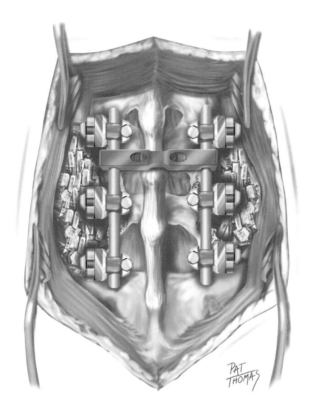

FIGURE 6-3E

Rods are placed. Bone graft is placed posterolaterally in the decorticated gutters.

Alternatively, a laminotomy can be performed so that the corresponding pedicle and lateral recess can be directly visualized or palpated with a nerve hook during insertion. Screw insertion is done in an analogous manner.

Once the hardware placement has been performed and the appropriate rods have been connected to the screws, the bone graft is placed into the decorticated gutters (Fig. 6–3E). Any laminotomy is covered with a fat graft or cellulose and a deep suction drain is placed. The muscles are returned to the midline and closed as a separate layer. In larger patients, a subcutaneous drain also may be placed.

POSTOPERATIVE CARE

The use of an orthosis is not indicated when interbody cages or segmental instrumentation are used. An orthosis has been thought by some to be associated with a lower incidence of graft collapse in the case of tricortical fusion. If the lumbosacral junction is fused, it is imperative to use an orthosis with a thigh cuff because a thoracolumbar sacral orthosis or chair back brace ending at the pelvis actually might increase joint reaction forces across L_5–S_1. If used, the orthosis is usually worn for 8 to 12 weeks.

OUTCOMES

Reported union rates for the interbody fusion using grafts have been in the area of 70% to 75%; initial data on the use of interbody cages suggests fusion rates as high as 92%. Posterolateral fusion rates with instrumentation are approximately 80% to 85%.

The outcomes in terms of pain relief are less predictable for axial pain syndromes than for compressive neurogenic pain syndromes. In one report, a good or excellent outcome was obtained by 46% of patients who underwent fusion for diskogenic low back pain. However, in the subset of patients who fused solidly, a clinical success rate of 96% was reported.

COMPLICATIONS

The main complication of interbody fusions without cages is graft subsidence and resultant neural foraminal stenosis. The incidence of this in the technically proficient arthrodesis, however, is quite low and approaches 8%. Subsidence of any significant degree has not been reported with cages; likewise, with the threaded cage design, back out has not been a problem. In males, anterior interbody fusion carries a risk of retrograde ejaculation of 0.5% due to injury of the hypogastric plexus.

With instrumented posterolateral fusion, the problems of potential hardware breakage and failure of fusion remain. The likelihood of hardware breakage is approximately one-half of 1%.

7

FRACTURES

- L$_2$ BURST FRACTURE WITH POSTERIOR SEGMENTAL INSTRUMENTATION
- L$_2$ BURST FRACTURE WITH ANTERIOR DECOMPRESSION AND INSTRUMENTED FUSION

- L$_2$ BURST FRACTURE WITH POSTERIOR SEGMENTAL INSTRUMENTATION

- L$_2$ BURST FRACTURE WITH ANTERIOR DECOMPRESSION AND INSTRUMENTED FUSION

SUMMARY

Fractures are classified into four major groups. The first category consists of compression fractures involving only the anterior column. The second category consists of burst fractures involving injury to the anterior and middle columns. The third category consists of injuries to all three biomechanical columns and is called an unstable burst fracture or fracture–dislocation. The fourth variety, a Chance fracture, is the result of a flexion vector. It is essentially a distraction injury to the middle and posterior columns with a compression injury anteriorly.

PRESENTATION

The compression fracture typically occurs in an osteoporotic individual. Local pain or radicular pain is the presenting symptom. The neurologic examination, as a rule, is normal.

The burst fracture is more severe, with flexion and compression vectors, with or without rotation, and involves injury to the anterior and middle columns. The radiographic hallmark of a burst fracture is widening of the interpedicular distance on the anteroposterior projection. This is a stable injury when only the anterior and middle columns are involved. Depending on retropulsion of fragments from the middle column encroaching on the spinal canal, neurologic deficit might be present.

An unstable burst fracture or fracture–dislocation involves an injury to all three columns. A particular variant of these, which involves a sagittal fracture in the spinous process, is frequently associated with neurologic deficit and a dural tear. Neurologic compromise can be minor or severe depending on the canal compromise.

The Chance fracture is caused by a flexion force and distraction of the middle and posterior columns. If this is predominantly a bony fracture, then the injury is stable with reduction. Because this is a canal-expanding lesion, the neurologic examination is usually normal. Due to the high association of Chance fractures with motor vehicle accidents involving flexion and rotation around a fixed pelvic fulcrum, intraabdominal injuries are common and must be ruled out.

NONOPERATIVE CARE

The compression fracture is treated nonoperatively. This involves reduction in a cast or a thoracolumbar sacral orthosis (TLSO). In general, orthotic therapy is not required for injuries resulting in less than 50% collapse.

The burst fracture involving the anterior and middle columns is a stable injury and can be treated by postural reduction and height maintenance in a TLSO. In more severe circumstances, where there is a greater degree of canal compromise, anterior decompression and stabilization might be indicated.

The unstable burst fracture, or fracture–dislocation, is not stable. It requires open reduction and internal fixation, which traditionally has been performed through a posterior approach. In the case of a neurologic deficit, all of these fractures should be imaged with CT to delineate the characteristics of the fracture and canal dimensions. In cases with greater than 40% canal compromise, posterior instrumentation should be applied to reduce this compromise. In a case of persistent neurologic deficit, postoperative CT myelography is indicated, with subsequent anterior decompression and fusion. Alternatively, with severe canal compromise and neurologic deficit, anterior decompression and fusion with instrumentation can be performed primarily.

The Chance fracture is stable if the fracture line traverses only bone. It can be treated by closed reduction and maintenance of lordosis or by open reduction and internal fixation with compression instrumentation. In those fractures that involve ligamentous injury or enter the disk space, a high rate of nonunion is to be expected; open reduction and internal fixation consisting of compression instrumentation and fusion is indicated.

DIAGNOSTIC STUDIES

Plain films are the initial test of choice. For injuries involving the middle or posterior columns (burst, unstable burst, or fracture–dislocation), widening of the pedicles will be seen on the anteroposterior view. CT is indicated for preoperative imaging of all of these injuries to determine the degree of canal compromise. If a decision is made to pursue posterior instrumentation with fracture reduction and attempt reduction of the fragments in the canal via ligamentotaxis, then postoperative CT myelography is frequently indicated; it is always indicated in the cases of persistent neurologic deficit.

PROCEDURES

L$_2$ BURST FRACTURE WITH POSTERIOR SEGMENTAL INSTRUMENTATION (FIG. 7–1)

In this example, the patient suffered a burst fracture and remained neurologically intact. The injury included the three columns. The principles of application of instrumentation include posterior distraction to restore disk height and appropriate contouring to restore segmental lordosis and kyphosis.

POSITIONING

The patient is intubated awake and transferred onto rolls on a padded frame, with the hips in extension (Fig. 7–1A). The patient is then asked to move the lower extremities on command. Once neurologic integrity has been confirmed, general anesthesia is induced. The use of somatosensory evoked potential monitoring is suggested. If this is not available, then a Stagnara wake-up test is mandatory after distraction and operative reduction of the fracture.

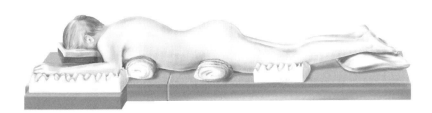

FIGURE 7–1A

L$_2$ BURST FRACTURE POSTERIOR SEGMENTAL INSTRUMEN-TATION. After awake intubation, the patient is positioned prone on rolls, with the hips in extension. Neurologic status is assessed, and general anesthesia is induced.

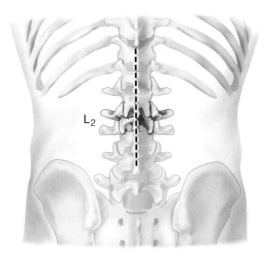

FIGURE 7–1B

An incision is made from T$_{11}$ to L$_4$, permitting exposure from T$_{12}$ to L$_3$.

TECHNIQUE

An incision is made in the skin from T$_{11}$ to L$_4$ (Fig. 7–1B). Hemostasis is obtained with electrocautery and self-retaining retractors are inserted. Dissection is carefully carried down toward the midline while observing the location of the hematoma. The hematoma alerts the surgeon to the location of the fracture and the resultant instability. The fascia is split on either side of the midline and a lateral spinal dissection is then carefully performed. Dissection is carried out to the transverse processes as well and decortication is performed (Fig. 7–1C). After hemostasis has been obtained, the position is confirmed with intraoperative radiography or fluoroscopy. The use of segmental instrumentation is left to the discretion of the surgeon, but it is generally recommended that the fracture be immobilized at least one segment below it and two above. Short segment fixation (e.g., in this case, pedicle screws placed at L$_1$ and L$_3$) has been associated with a high rate of subsequent kyphotic collapse when anterior column support is not applied as an adjunct.

In the present example, a claw construct consisting of hooks is applied from T$_{12}$ to L$_1$. Hooks are upgoing under the pedicles at L$_1$, with a downgoing transverse process hook and laminar hook at T$_{12}$. These are then compressed. Interpedicular screws are placed at L$_3$. The canal may be opened, if desired, to palpate the lateral recess. If not, a point lateral to the facet bisecting the midpoint of the transverse process over the L$_3$ pedicle is chosen. The cortex is broached with a small high-speed burr and the pedicle is probed. This tract is then tapped and filled with the appropriate length screw. The position should be checked with static x-ray or intraoperative fluoroscopy.

Rods are then cut and contoured to accommodate the segmental lordosis. These are then applied to the hardware in a sequential fashion (Fig. 7–1D). The segment between L$_1$ and L$_3$ is then distracted to reduce the fracture. Derotation maneuvers also can be used to further reconstitute the lordosis. Once reduction is confirmed by x-ray, a wake-up test is performed if evoked potential monitoring is not available.

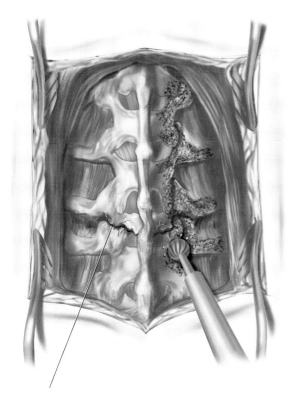

Fracture at L_2

FIGURE 7-1C

A wide exposure is made to the tips of the transverse processes from T_{11} to L_3. Decortication of the entire posterior surface including laminae and transverse processes is performed. The fractured lamina at L_2 should be decorticated gently, if at all.

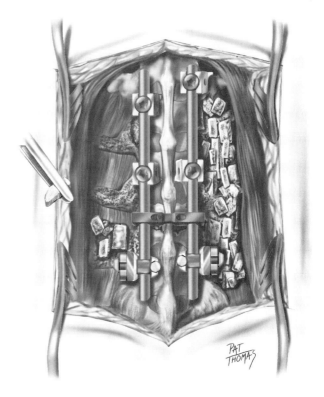

FIGURE 7-1D

Fixation at two levels rostral and one level caudal to the fracture is recommended. A claw construct using hooks is preferred at T_{12}–L_1. Interpedicular fixation is placed at L_3. A two-rod construct with cross-linking is assembled. Bone graft is placed on all decorticated surfaces.

The bone graft is then harvested by a separate incision over the iliac crest. This is done in the standard manner and the wound is closed over a drain. The posterior elements from T_{12} to L_3 along with the transverse processes of L_1, L_2, and L_3 are decorticated and the gutters are packed with bone graft. The graft is also placed posteriorly from T_{12} to L_3. A cross-link can be applied, if so desired.

The wound is then irrigated and closed over a suction drain. The muscles are returned to the midline and the fascia is repaired. A second subcutaneous drain may be in order.

L_2 BURST FRACTURE WITH ANTERIOR DECOMPRESSION AND INSTRUMENTED FUSION (FIG. 7–2)

An alternative approach, particularly in cases of severe canal compromise, is anterior decompression and reconstruction. The use of anterior instrumentation, in many cases, also has obviated a secondary or staged posterior procedure.

POSITIONING

In the present example, after awake intubation, the patient is transferred to the operating table and placed in a left-side-up, lateral decubitus position (Fig. 7–2A). Somatosensory evoked potential monitoring is required; if this is not available, a Stagnara wake-up test should be performed when the fracture has been reduced. An axillary roll is placed and padded supports such as bean bags or towels are placed to ensure that the patient is perpendicular to the floor of the operating room in the lateral decubitus position. Bony prominences, including the fibular head and the tibial plateaus, also must be meticulously padded.

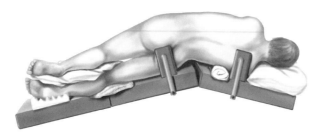

FIGURE 7–2A

L_2 BURST FRACTURE ANTERIOR DECOMPRESSION AND INSTRUMENTED FUSION. After awake intubation, the patient is transferred to the operating table and placed in a left-side up, lateral decubitus position. An axillary roll is placed and bony prominences are padded. The table can be jack-knifed.

TECHNIQUE

A T_{10} thoracotomy is then performed. An incision is made over the tenth rib and dissection is carried through the latissimus dorsi to the periosteal surface (Fig. 7–2B). The periosteum is incised directly on the rib head and a periosteal elevator is used to isolate that. Care must be taken to isolate the neurovascular bundle inferiorly. The rib is then cut anteriorly and posteriorly as far as possible and saved for graft. The left lung is deflated and dissection is carried down to the L_2 body. The iliopsoas must be reflected carefully to avoid injury to the overlying genitofemoral nerve. Overlying soft tissue is reflected and segmental vessels are ligated and dissected posteriorly. In this way, the entire expanse from L_1 to L_3 is exposed (Fig. 7–2C).

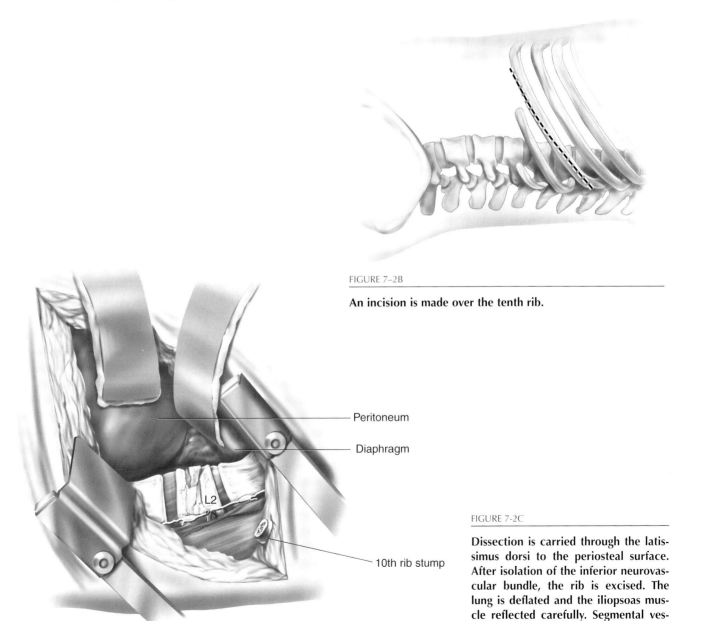

FIGURE 7–2B

An incision is made over the tenth rib.

Peritoneum

Diaphragm

L2

10th rib stump

FIGURE 7-2C

Dissection is carried through the latissimus dorsi to the periosteal surface. After isolation of the inferior neurovascular bundle, the rib is excised. The lung is deflated and the iliopsoas muscle reflected carefully. Segmental vessels are ligated.

A decompression is then performed at L_2 (Fig. 7–2D). This may be a complete corpectomy in the case of severe injury or posterior decompression if the remaining anterior column support is structurally useful. In cases of complete corpectomy, discs are removed completely at L_{1-2} and L_{2-3}, with curettage back to the bleeding bone of the rostral L_1 and caudal L_3 end-plates.

After corpectomy and hemostasis with bipolar electrocautery, transverse screws are placed in the bodies of L_1 and L_3. This should be done under fluoroscopic guidance or verified with planar films. The screw should be placed as far posteriorly as possible and parallel to the spinal canal. An awl is used to broach the cortex and the screws are inserted. Bicortical purchase is preferred. After placement of screws at L_1 and L_3, distraction is performed. The interbody graft is then placed; the graft can consist of a tricortical iliac crest graft, fibular allograft augmented with rib autograft, or titanium mesh cage filled with autograft or allograft. Once the graft is placed, the distraction device is removed and instrumentation is placed. Derotation screws are then placed through the plate in an analogous manner (Fig. 7–2E).

The wound is then copiously irrigated and, if evoked potential monitoring is not available, a wake-test is performed.

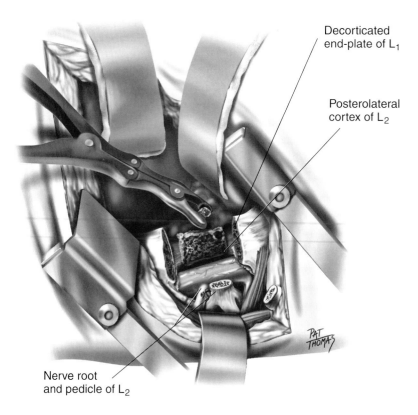

Decorticated
end-plate of L_1

Posterolateral
cortex of L_2

Nerve root
and pedicle of L_2

FIGURE 7-2D

Decompression is performed at L_2, which can be a complete corpectomy or posterior decompression only.

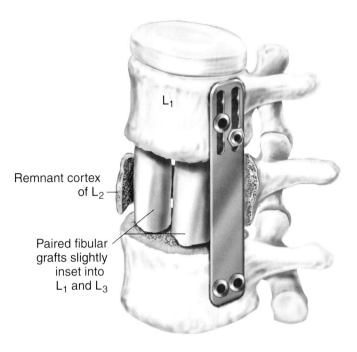

Remnant cortex
of L$_2$

Paired fibular
grafts slightly
inset into
L$_1$ and L$_3$

FIGURE 7-2E

Transverse screws are placed in the bodies of L$_1$ and L$_3$ and verified fluoroscopically. Bicortical purchase is preferred. The segment is distracted, grafts are placed, and the instrumentation assembled.

The wound is then closed in layers. The diaphragm does not need to be repaired per se, although this is preferable if a margin is available. A thoracostomy tube is placed and brought out several interspaces from the wound. The wound is then closed in layers with approximation of the ninth and eleventh ribs, followed by subcutaneous and skin closure.

POSTOPERATIVE CARE

Patients are maintained in a TLSO for 6 to 12 weeks. Ambulation is encouraged as soon as possible postoperatively.

OUTCOMES

The expected union rate is quite high for anterior and posterior procedures and exceeds 85%. The rate of neurologic recovery depends on the severity of injury; in the case of injuries involving the cauda equina, the prognosis for neurologic recovery is excellent. In any patient who has incomplete neurologic injury, consideration should be given to intravenous methylprednisolone within 8 hours of injury; therapy consists of 30 mg/kg of methylprednisolone given over 1 hour followed by 5.4 mg/kg per hour for the subsequent 23 hours.

COMPLICATIONS

Complications are nonunion, hardware failure, and persistent neurologic deficit after initial attempts at reduction. In those patients with persistent neurologic deficits, myelography followed by axial CT should be performed within 5 to 7 days after the procedure. In cases of residual or continuing compression, additional decompressive or stabilization procedures may be required.

8

TUMORS

- L$_2$ TUMOR–POSTERIOR SEGMENTAL INSTRUMENTATION
- ANTERIOR DECOMPRESSION AND FUSION

- L$_2$ TUMOR–POSTERIOR SEGMENTAL INSTRUMENTATION

- ANTERIOR DECOMPRESSION AND FUSION

SUMMARY

The most common tumor in the spine is metastatic. Frequent sources of primary neoplasms are breast, lung, thyroid, kidney, and prostate. The most common primary bone-forming malignancy in the spine is osteosarcoma, although this is comparatively rare. The most common primary malignancy in the spine is myeloma or plasmocytoma. In general, the prognosis differs depending on the tumor type, dissemination at presentation, and local features. Overall, for metastatic disease of the spine, median survival is 2 years.

The most common classification scheme involving spinal tumors is that of Harrington. It is based on structural features and neurologic examination and is largely independent of tissue type or prognosis. In Harrington class I, metastatic disease of the spine is present. The neurologic examination is intact and no deformity is present. In class II, there is bony involvement, clearly evident in plain films, but without collapse or neurologic alteration. In class III, the disease is limited to the neural elements and structural integrity is the rule. Neurologic impairment, however, might be present. In general, classes I through III are treated nonoperatively with radiation or adjuvant chemotherapy. The treatment of class IV and V patients is usually surgical in nature. In class IV, bony destruction and kyphosis are present. In class V, bony destruction, kyphosis, and neurologic encroachment and impairment are present.

Benign tumors include osteoid osteoma, which commonly presents as painful scoliosis in adolescence, aneurysmal bone cyst, giant cell tumor, osteochondroma, eosinophilic granuloma, and hemangioma. Of these, the most ominous is giant cell tumor. There is a 5% to 15% risk of sarcomatous degeneration in giant cell tumors that have been treated with radiation therapy. In contrast, hemangioma is a very common, incidental finding seen in up to 10% of asymptomatic individuals.

PRESENTATION

Most spine tumors, benign or malignant, present with local axial pain. Neurologic involvement is uncommon as a primary presenting symptom. Atypical mechanical features such as night pain should alert the clinician to the possibility of neoplasia. In addition, certain specific features such as response to aspirin suggest a particular lesion (osteoid osteoma). The presence of constitutional symptoms would further alert the clinician to the possibility of tumor. It should be recalled that up to 10% of patients with an unknown primary tumor present with back pain due to metastatic disease as their first symptom. This most commonly occurs in individuals older than 50 years.

NONOPERATIVE CARE

For benign tumors, in the absence of pathologic fracture or deformity, supportive care is the rule. This can consist of orthotic wear, analgesics, or nonsteroidal drugs. For more locally aggressive tumors such as giant cell or hemangioma, low dose radiation may be beneficial.

For pathologic compression fractures due to benign tumors, orthotic support is indicated. This may or may not be coupled with low dose radiation depending on the lesion. For metastatic disease, Harrington classes I through III, radiation therapy and chemotherapy are typically effective. Likewise, for myeloma or plasmocytoma, radiation is the mainstay of treatment.

DIAGNOSTIC STUDIES

When a lytic lesion is seen on plain films, approximately 30% of the volume of the vertebral body will have been affected. MRI is by far the most sensitive tool for determining occult lesions, and it is a valuable tool for imaging the degree of axial involvement, collapse, and canal compression. CT myelography might be beneficial in further delineating bony compression, and bone scan is valuable for determining the extent of skeletal involvement. Certain tumors, however, specifically eosinophilic granuloma, myeloma, metastatic thyroid carcinoma, and metastatic renal cell carcinoma, might be "cold" on a bone scan. Obviously, serum protein electrophoresis is valuable in making the diagnosis of myeloma; in up to 20% of people, the only abnormality might be a urine gamma-globulin spike.

The patient presenting with a spinal lesion and unknown primary tumor represents a diagnostic challenge. In general, the lesion should be biopsied only as a last resort because the recovery of tissue from these specimens yields a firm tissue diagnosis in only 60% to 70% of cases. All efforts should be directed at finding the primary lesion. This is best done by a combination of CT scanning of the chest and abdomen, serum protein electrophoresis, and, where indicated, prostate-specific antigen. With this approach, the primary tumor should be discovered in more than 80% of the cases.

In the case of metastatic disease with a progressive kyphotic deformity, neurologic deterioration or compromise, or resistance to adjuvant therapy, anterior decompression with fusion, with or without supplementary posterior stabilization, is usually indicated. In comparatively rare cases such as a metastatic renal cell carcinoma, which can involve the posterior elements only, posterior stabilization alone might be sufficient. In the case of primary bone tumors, where a marginal excision is indicated to prevent local recurrence, spondylectomy or partial vertebrectomy is indicated.

PROCEDURES

L$_2$ TUMOR – POSTERIOR SEGMENTAL INSTRUMENTATION (FIG. 8–1)

POSITIONING AND TECHNIQUE

The patient is positioned on an extension frame, with the pelvis minimally flexed and the legs in neutral (Fig. 8–1A). Slight hip and knee flexion usually is required. All bony prominences are padded thoroughly, and the lumbar spine is then prepared and draped into a sterile field. Care must be taken during prepping and draping to leave the iliac crests exposed for bone graft harvest.

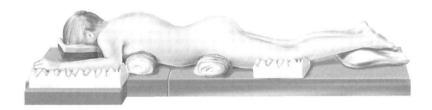

FIGURE 8–1A

L$_2$ TUMOR—POSTERIOR SEGMENTAL INSTRUMENTATION. The patient is positioned on an extension frame, with the pelvis minimally flexed and the legs in neutral. Bony prominences are padded thoroughly.

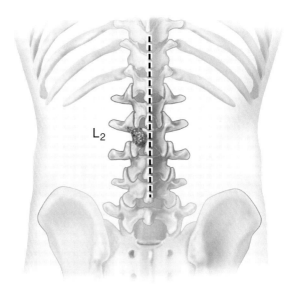

FIGURE 8–1B

An incision is made from T$_{11}$ to L$_4$.

An incision is made in the posterior elements from T$_{11}$ to L$_4$ (Fig. 8–1B). Fluoroscopy or static x-ray can be used to localize the appropriate levels before skin incision. A standard posterior approach is then performed, with dissection down to the fascia. Incision of the fascia on either side of the midline and a careful lateral subperiosteal stripping are performed. Muscles are reflected out to the facets. At this point, a self-retaining retractor system is inserted and a far lateral dissection follows, with stripping of the deep layers of the paraspinous muscle, including the multifidus, to expose the lamina and transverse processes of T$_{12}$, L$_1$, L$_2$, and L$_3$. During the approach, care must be taken when approaching the lesion. Bone quality is frequently suboptimal and inadvertent neurologic injury could result from overzealous muscle stripping (Fig. 8–1C).

The tumor is then removed. Frequently, laminotomy is required at the rostral and caudal edges of the involved level, with the lamina, facet, and pars removed in order to allow resection of the tumor (Fig. 8–1D).

After decompression, the iliac crest bone graft is harvested in the standard manner. A curvilinear incision is made over the posterior iliac crest at the level of the posterosuperior iliac spine (PSIS). Dissection is carried down to the gluteal fascia, which is incised on the iliac crest. Self-retaining retractors are inserted and the fascia is stripped from the dorsal aspect of the crest and the lateral table. The gluteus medius is reflected with electrocautery, and a Taylor retractor is inserted to reflect the gluteus. Care should be taken to dissect directly anteriorly from the PSIS because of the location of the sciatic notch. The sciatic notch can be routinely palpated once gluteal stripping has been accomplished. Gouges and osteotomes are then used to harvest multiple cortical and cancellous strips of bone for grafting.

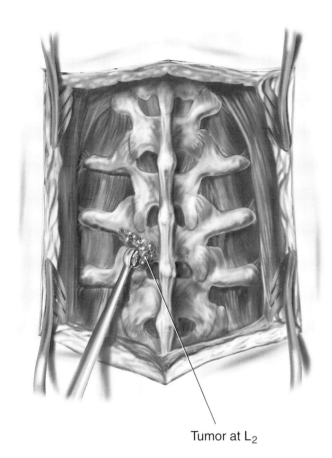

Tumor at L$_2$

FIGURE 8-1C

Wide exposure is performed. The lamina and transverse processes of T$_{12}$, L$_1$, L$_2$, and L$_3$ should be clearly visualized. Care must be taken when approaching the lesion because bone quality is usually compromised. The tumor is then resected. Posterior elements are decorticated.

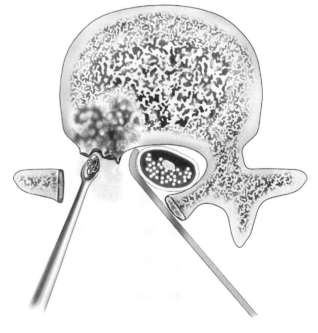

FIGURE 8-1D

Posterolateral fusion is performed with bone graft from T$_{12}$ to L$_3$.

Posterolateral fusion is then performed. The lamina of T_{12}, the transverse processes of L_1, L_2, and L_3, and the corresponding aspects of the lateral zygapophyseal joints are decorticated. The harvested bone is placed into the trough created on either side of the spine.

Internal fixation is then placed by using interpedicular segmental fixation at L_3 and a claw construct at T_{12}–L_1 (Fig. 8–1E). Screw insertion can be done with the open or closed technique. In the open technique, laminotomies are made at L_2–L_3 to expose the L_3 pedicles. With a nerve hook or probe in the lateral recess to reflect the corresponding root medially, the pedicle is entered with an awl or a drill and, under direct vision, cannulated. Screw insertion should be checked with static films or fluoroscopy. Landmarks for entry of the pedicle are found by dividing the corresponding transverse process in half in a rostral-to-caudal direction and then extending this line to the lateral margin of the facet. This so-called far lateral approach affords the additional advantage of sparing the facet capsule. The claw is constructed as follows: upgoing pedicle hooks bilaterally at L_1 with unilateral downgoing laminar and transverse process hooks at T_{12}. After insertion of screws and hooks, appropriate rods are placed.

A drain is placed in the depths of each wound, which are closed in layers. Fascia, subcutaneous tissue, and skin must be closed separately, followed by compressive dressings.

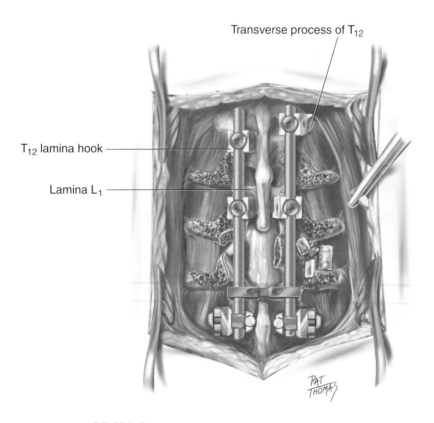

Transverse process of T_{12}

T_{12} lamina hook

Lamina L_1

FIGURE 8–1E

Internal fixation is then placed, with interpedicular fixation at L_3 and a claw construct at T_{12}-L_1.

Intraoperative spinal cord monitoring can be beneficial in these cases, particularly if correction of a deformity is involved. It should be borne in mind that somatosensory evoked potential monitoring assesses only the function of the dorsal sensory columns and provides no information concerning the involvement of motor columns. If this is a concern, the supplementary Stagnara wake-up test must be performed. If motor evoked potential monitoring is available, the wake-up test is not necessary.

In the case of a patient with anterior column involvement (as is the case 90% of the time with metastatic disease), corpectomy and reconstruction are indicated.

ANTERIOR DECOMPRESSION AND FUSION (FIG. 8–2)

POSITIONING

A patient with an L_2 metastatic lesion is placed in the lateral decubitus position, with all bony prominences padded (Fig. 8–2A). This is best afforded by a beanbag or kidney rests. In general, the patient should be positioned so that there is no lateral tilt, i.e., the patient is perpendicular to the operating table. This position provides the surgeon greater flexibility with anatomic landmarks for decompression and subsequent reconstruction.

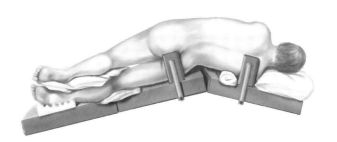

FIGURE 8–2A

ANTERIOR DECOMPRESSION AND FUSION. The patient is placed in lateral decubitus position, with all bony prominences padded.

TECHNIQUE

A T_{10} thoracotomy is then performed. An incision is made over the tenth rib and dissection is carried down through the soft tissue planes to the rib (Fig. 8–2B). The latis-

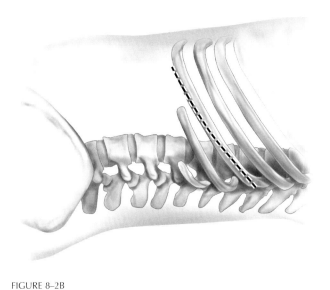

FIGURE 8–2B

An incision is made over the tenth rib.

simus dorsi is reflected posteriorly. The periosteum over the rib is incised, and, while taking care to protect the neurovascular bundle, the rib is harvested as far posteriorly as possible. That tissue should be saved for later use as graft material.

The lung is then deflated and reflected anteriorly. The L_2 level is then localized by x-ray and direct visualization. The overlying tissue is reflected and control of segmental vessels is obtained. A complete lateral exposure, including reflection of the iliopsoas, is then performed to visualize L_1, L_2, and L_3.

Corpectomy is then performed by incising the disk spaces of L_1–L_2 and L_3–L_4. Curettes and rongeurs are used to resect L_2 completely (Fig. 8–2C). An alternative technique is that of spondylectomy. In this technique, the bases of the pedicles are divided with a Gigli saw or a Kerrison rongeur, the posterior margin of the vertebra is gently reflected anteriorly, and, after division of the other pedicle, the body is removed en bloc. This is a demanding technique and should be reserved for cases where en bloc resection directly affects the patient's survival, e.g., localized contained osteosarcoma.

After complete corpectomy and visualization of the posterior longitudinal ligament, bipolar electrocautery is used to control epidural bleeding. Thrombin-soaked methylcellulose may be required for packing. Disks are completely removed and end-plates at L_1 and L_3 are curetted back to the bleeding bone. Care should be taken not to enter the end-plates or inadvertently resect normal bone at adjacent levels.

Fibular allograft, rib allograft, or a titanium mesh cage can be used for anterior column support (Fig. 8–2D). The titanium mesh cage, which has been shown to be as rigid as an allograft in laboratory tests, can be packed with crushed, cortical cancellous bone or allograft. Alternatively, an autograft can be cut to an appropriate length and inserted between the levels to be fused. In this case, it would be firmly anchored in the endplates of L_1 and L_3. Supplementary anterior fixation in the form of a lateral plate device is added. In certain cases, with the integrity of posterior elements preserved, the entire procedure can be performed anteriorly.

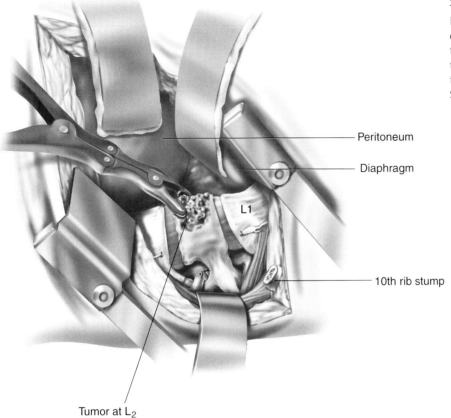

FIGURE 8-2C

Dissection is carried through the latissimus dorsi to the periosteal surface. After isolation of the inferior neurovascular bundle, the rib is excised. The lung is deflated and the iliopsoas muscle is carefully reflected. Segmental vessels are ligated.

—— Peritoneum

—— Diaphragm

—— 10th rib stump

L1

Tumor at L_2

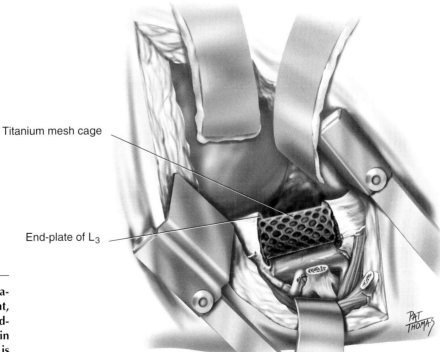

Titanium mesh cage

End-plate of L_3

FIGURE 8-2D

After complete corpectomy and visualization of the posterior longitudinal ligament, epidural bleeding is controlled and endplates are prepared. An anterior support, in this instance, a titanium mesh cage, is inserted. Supplementary anterior fixation is added.

Ribs should be approximated with a heavy, absorbable suture. The wound is then closed in layers over a thoracostomy tube.

POSTOPERATIVE CARE

These patients are supported in an orthosis (TLSO) for 8 to 12 weeks. If adjuvant radiation therapy is contemplated, it should be delayed for at least 3 weeks. This period allows the soft tissue to heal and does not compromise the eventual integrity of the fusion mass.

OUTCOMES

The goal of surgery for spinal tumors is to reverse or prevent progressive deformity, address neurologic compression, and alleviate pain. The union rate for fusion is comparable to that in other procedures in the absence of steroid therapy or injudicious radiation. The success of neurologic decompression depends on the extent of neurologic deficit at the time of presentation; lesions compressing the cauda equina have a prognosis superior to those in the thoracic and cervical spine. The outcome regarding pain relief is excellent, with most patients reporting dramatic relief from their pain after surgery.

COMPLICATIONS

Persistent complications are delayed wound healing and non-union of the graft in the setting of postoperative radiation. In general, the incidence of infection is comparable to that of elective cases. In patients with short life expectancies (less than 6 months), in whom the surgery is palliative, polymethylmethacrylate can be considered as a reconstructive material. This affords immediate stability and pain relief. However, polymethylmethacrylate will loosen over time and, as such, should not be used in patients with longer life expectancies.

9

INFECTION

- CORPECTOMY AND INTERBODY FUSION (L$_2$)
- DRAINAGE OF EPIDURAL ABSCESS

- CORPECTOMY AND INTERBODY FUSION (L$_2$)

- DRAINAGE OF EPIDURAL ABSCESS

SUMMARY

Spinal infections can involve bony structures (osteomyelitis or tuberculous spondylitis) or the epidural space. An epidural abscess is a surgical emergency. Most bony infections are anterior (vertebral body) because of the arrangement of Batson's valveless plexus. Primary diskitis is uncommon after childhood because of the closure of the vessels supplying the intervertebral disk. In an adult, diskitis is almost always secondary to external inoculation. In general, with the exception of epidural abscess, the treatment of a spinal infection is medical once the appropriate microbial diagnosis has been made. Treatment consists of prolonged intravenous antibiotics with or without orthotic support. Should the patient not respond to antibiotics or exhibit sequestration, progressive deformity, or neurologic deterioration, then surgical debridement and reconstruction are required. In the case of a significant epidural abscess, surgical evacuation is the rule. It should be borne in mind that in this section spinal infections will be discussed as *osteomyelitis*; the principles of surgical management for osteomyelitis are very similar to those used for tuberculous spondylitis.

PRESENTATION

Clinical presentation is highly variable. A high index of suspicion is essential. Back pain is uniformly present. This pain is frequently atypical in that it can be experienced at night or when recumbent. The pain is usually unrelated to activities. Approximately half of the patients have constitutional symptoms such as malaise and fever. Neurologic findings are present in approximately 5% of patients at presentation. Physical examination is non-specific. The involved area might be tender to palpation with associated muscle spasm. Very few patients will have signs of meningeal irritation.

Epidural abscess formation is rare, with an incidence of approximately 3%. Predisposing factors are advanced age (seventh decade), diabetes, immunosuppression, alcohol abuse, and a history of invasive procedures. Initially, patients present with back pain accompanied by constitutional signs of infection. This typically leads to radicular pain and neurologic deficit. Overall, the mortality rate is approximately 15%. The rate of neurologic deterioration can be quite rapid, i.e., between 48 and 72 hours. The most frequent location of epidural abscess formation is the lumbar spine, followed by the thoracic spine.

NONOPERATIVE CARE

In the majority of cases, vertebral osteomyelitis is caused by *Staphylococcus aureus*. Once the organism has been identified via biopsy, treatment consists of 6 to 12 weeks of intravenous antibiotics. Closed-needle biopsies will successfully identify an organism approximately 70% of the time, whereas open biopsies will correctly identify a microbe 80% to 90% of the time. Depending on the extent of the infection, an orthosis might be appropriate during the course of antimicrobial therapy.

The conservative care of granulomatous spondylitis also involves chemotherapy. This usually consists of a four-drug regimen (isoniazid, rifampin, ethambutol, and pyrazinamide). Medical treatment is continued for 6 to 12 months.

There is no nonoperative treatment for epidural abscess. Once MRI has identified the abscess, emergent laminectomy for drainage is indicated.

DIAGNOSTIC STUDIES

In cases of osteomyelitis, the erythrocyte sedimentation rate and C-reactive protein level are elevated. Blood cultures are positive in approximately three-fourths of the patients. Radionuclide imaging is indicated. Gallium scans in conjunction with technetium scans have been reported to an accuracy of 90%. Indium 111 scans have been used, but are handicapped by a high false negative rate. CT is helpful only in delineating bony margins or guiding a needle biopsy. MRI is the test of choice. Osteomyelitis can be identified by a characteristic pattern of changes on MRI, with decreased T1-weighted intensity in the vertebral body and disk and an indistinct margin between the two. There also is increased signal intensity in T2-weighted sequences in the vertebral body and disk.

Likewise, for epidural abscess, MRI is the diagnostic modality of choice. It is superior to CT myelography in its ability to provide information on the consistency of the extrinsic mass compressing the neural elements.

PROCEDURES

CORPECTOMY AND INTERBODY FUSION (L$_2$) (FIG. 9–1)

POSITIONING AND TECHNIQUE

In the case of a patient with vertebral osteomyelitis, corpectomy and reconstruction are indicated. The patient with an L$_2$ lesion is positioned in the lateral decubitus position, with all bony prominences padded (Fig. 9–1A). This is best afforded by a beanbag or kidney rests. In general, the patient should be positioned so that there is no lateral tilt, i.e., the patient is perpendicular to the operating table. This allows the surgeon greater flexibility with anatomic landmarks for decompression and subsequent reconstruction. A T$_{10}$ thoracotomy is then performed. An incision is made over the tenth rib and dissection is carried down through the soft tissue planes to the rib (Fig. 9–1B). The latissimus dorsi is reflected posteriorly. The periosteum over the rib

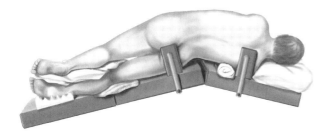

FIGURE 9–1A

INFECTION—CORPECTOMY AND INTERBODY FUSION (L$_2$). The patient is placed in a lateral decubitus position, with all bony prominences padded.

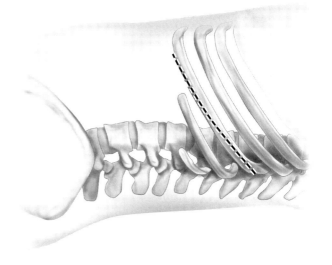

FIGURE 9–1B

An incision is made over the tenth rib.

is incised, and, while taking care to protect the neurovascular bundle, the rib is harvested as far posteriorly as possible. The harvested tissue should be saved for later use as graft material.

The lung is deflated and reflected anteriorly. The L_2 level is then localized by x-ray and direct visualization. The overlying tissue is reflected and control of segmental vessels is obtained. A complete lateral exposure, including reflection of the iliopsoas, is then performed to visualize L_1, L_2, and L_3 (Fig. 9–1C). Corpectomy is then performed by incising the disk spaces of L_1–L_2 and L_3–L_4. Curettes and rongeurs are used to resect L_2 completely (Fig. 9–1D).

After complete corpectomy and visualization of the posterior longitudinal ligament, bipolar electrocautery is used to control epidural bleeding. Thrombin-soaked methylcellulose might be required for packing. Disks are completely removed and end-plates at L_1 and L_3 are curetted back to the bleeding bone. Care should be taken not to enter the end-plates or inadvertently resect normal bone at the adjacent levels.

Fibular allograft, rib allograft, or titanium mesh cage can be used for anterior column support. The titanium mesh cage, which has been shown to be as rigid as an allo-

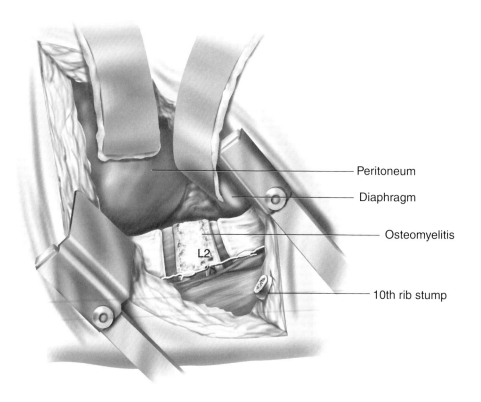

FIGURE 9-1C

Dissection is carried through the latissimus dorsi to the periosteal surface. After isolation of the inferior neurovascular bundle, the rib is excised. The lung is deflated and the iliopsoas muscle is carefully reflected. Segmental vessels are ligated.

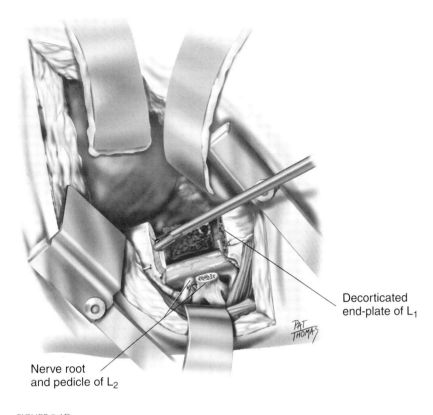

Decorticated
end-plate of L$_1$

Nerve root
and pedicle of L$_2$

FIGURE 9-1D

**A complete corpectomy is performed at L$_2$. L$_1$ and L$_3$ end-
plates are prepared.**

graft in laboratory tests, can be packed with crushed, cortical cancellous bone or
allograft. Alternatively, an autograft can be cut to an appropriate length and inserted
between the levels to be fused. In this case, it would be firmly anchored in the end-
plates of L$_1$ and L$_3$.

Before inserting grafting material, a thorough debridement of all necrotic or
infected material is mandatory. This would include end-plates, disk material, and soft
tissue. The epidural space should be meticulously debrided. If the infection involves
more than one level, all levels should be examined at the time of the initial procedure, even at the risk of extending the decompression and fusion.

Grafting can be done primarily if a meticulous debridement has been performed. The primary addition of anterior instrumentation can increase the risk of
recurrent infection, but currently there are no firm data on this (Fig. 9–1E).

Ribs should be approximated with a heavy, absorbable suture. The wound is
then closed in layers over a thoracostomy tube.

If anterior instrumentation is not used, consideration should be given to a
delayed posterior stabilization procedure with instrumentation. This should be
delayed 1 to 2 weeks to avoid the possibility of bacteremic seeding of the posterior
surgical site.

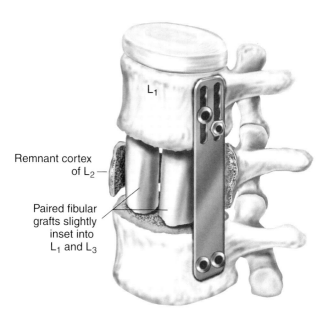

FIGURE 9-1E

Interbody graft is placed after thorough debridement of all necrotic tissue. Grafting can be done primarily if meticulous debridement has been performed. Anterior instrumentation may be added, but doing so may increase the risk of recurrent infection.

DRAINAGE OF EPIDURAL ABSCESS (FIG. 9–2)

POSITIONING AND TECHNIQUE

The patient is placed prone in the knee-to-chest position or on rolls. All extremities are padded (Fig. 9–2A). A standard midline approach is made over the involved area

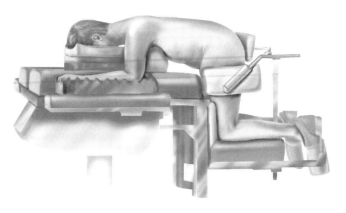

FIGURE 9–2A

DRAINAGE OF EPIDURAL ABSCESS. The patient is placed prone in the knee-to-chest position.

(Fig. 9–2B). Dissection is carried through the subcutaneous tissue to the fascia, which is split on either side of the midline. Dissection is carried out laterally to the facets. Self-retaining retractors are inserted, and laminotomy is performed in a standard way. The ligamentum flavum is elevated with a curette. It can be resected sharply and the epidural space palpated with a nerve hook. Laminectomy is then performed with a Kerrison rongeur until the purulent material is drained (Fig. 9–2C). The canal should be inspected for any residual material. The wound is then copiously irrigated.

The fascia, subcutaneous tissue, and skin are then closed in layers over a suction drain (Fig. 9–2D).

FIGURE 9–2B

A midline incision is made over the involved level.

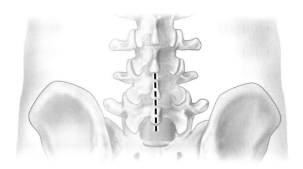

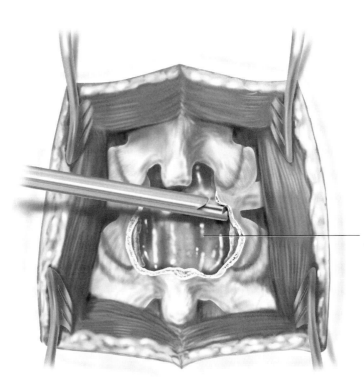

Purulent material to be drained

FIGURE 9-2C

The fascia is split in the midline and dissection is carried laterally to the facets. A standard laminotomy is performed and ligamentum flavum is elevated with a curette. This process is continued until purulent material is encountered.

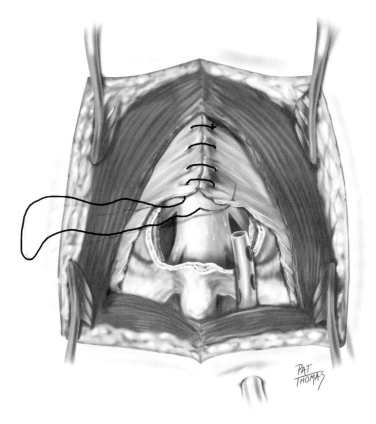

FIGURE 9-2D

Purulent material is drained and the wound is copiously irrigated. Closure is performed over a suction drain.

POSTOPERATIVE CARE

Patients undergoing anterior corpectomy should be supported postoperatively with a TLSO. The patient is mobilized after removal of the drains.

In the case of drainage of an epidural abscess, the patient is mobilized as soon as possible. The suction drain should be left in place until the drainage is minimal. Intravenous antibiotics should be continued for approximately 4 to 6 weeks.

OUTCOMES

Osteomyelitis/tuberculous spondylitis   In general, the fusion rate for anterior corpectomy with primary instrumentation or secondary posterior instrumentation is in excess of 90%. The outlook for eradication of disease is excellent, assuming a thorough surgical debridement, adequate antimicrobial diagnosis, and 6 to 8-weeks of intravenous antibiotics.

Epidural abscess   The outcome of laminectomy for epidural abscess depends largely on the presentation and swiftness of diagnosis. The prognosis is good provided the abscess is promptly recognized and drained. Poor prognosis is associated with rapidly ascending neurologic deficit including paralysis or deficits present for 36 to 48 hours. Other negative prognostic factors are diabetes, immunosuppression, and advanced age.

COMPLICATIONS

Risks of hardware failure and non-union approximate those in fracture care assuming a thorough debridement has been accomplished. Complications from epidural abscess include persistent neurologic deficit. Overall mortality, despite timely intervention and appropriate antimicrobial therapy, remains at 10% to 15%.

PART II

THORACIC SPINE

10

DISK HERNIATION

- ## POSTEROLATERAL DISK EXCISION
- ## ANTERIOR DISK EXCISION

- ## POSTEROLATERAL DISK EXCISION

SUMMARY

Thoracic disk herniations can result in myelopathic syndromes at the thoracic spinal cord level. On occasion, isolated radicular symptoms can arise related to lateral disk herniations involving the thoracic nerve roots. Thoracic diskectomies account for approximately one-half of 1% of all diskectomy operations, although the incidence of asymptomatic disk herniation based on necropsy and imaging studies can be as high as 10% to 15%.

Surgery is generally not indicated for these conditions; it is reserved for myelopathy from spinal cord compression. The decision as to whether to perform surgery from an anterior or posterior approach is related to the clinical symptoms and the imaging studies that indicate the location of the disk herniation. Posterolateral disk excision might be indicated for patients who have unilateral symptoms and disk herniation not extending beyond the midline. Calcification of the disk, which is common in thoracic disk herniations, might be an indication to proceed with an anterior rather than a posterolateral approach. The spinal cord should never be retracted during performance of this procedure because of risk for neurologic injury.

For the isolated disk herniation, the most common location is central or central–lateral, accounting for 60% to 80%. The most commonly involved level is T_{11-12}. Three-fourths of the herniations occur in the lower thoracic spine, between T_8 and T_{11}.

PRESENTATION

In the patient with a large central disk herniation resulting in canal stenosis, thoracic myelopathy can result. The myelopathy presents as a combination of intercostal neuritis with pain and sensory changes in the involved dermatome. Distal hyperreflexia and upper motor neuron signs accompany it. In the case of a pure lateral disk herniation with intraforaminal extension, intercostal pain is present without distal upper motor neuron signs. Atypical radiating pains also can occur to the groin and testes. Chest and/or abdominal pain also might be present, depending on the level of the prolapse. In the caudal cervical spine, neck pain and axillary pain (secondary to T_1 irritation) might be present. Such pain also might be associated with Horner's syndrome (ipsilateral ptosis, myosis, and anhydrosis).

More than one-half of patients have motor and sensory findings at the time of presentation. Up to one-third of the patients might have genitourinary (GU) or gastrointestinal (GI) dysfunction associated with myelopathic symptoms. Neurologic deterioration is rare because of the chronic nature of these problems. Surgery is based on the degree of functional incapacity.

NONOPERATIVE CARE

A brief period of bed rest, anti-inflammatory medications, and analgesics might be indicated. The use of an orthosis is controversial. The efficacy of physical therapy has not been proven. Oral or epidural steroid therapy has not been shown to be effective in this region.

DIAGNOSTIC STUDIES

Plain radiographs might show calcification of the posterior aspects of the annulus fibrosus. Sagittal alignment also is important. Patients with kyphosis are more prone to neurologic problems due to thoracic disk herniations. Instability is uncommon. MRI is the imaging procedure of choice to assess the extent of the herniation, abnormalities related to cord compression, or parenchymal changes within the spinal cord. Myelogram with CT also can be useful but generally has been supplanted by MRI.

PROCEDURE

POSTEROLATERAL DISK EXCISION (FIG. 10–1)

POSITIONING

The patient is positioned prone (Fig. 10–1A). The chest and pelvis are supported on rolls. The correct level is identified by palpation of the ribs and radiographic confirmation.

TECHNIQUE

The spine is approached laterally. The cord should not be retracted.

Posterolateral access is gained through the proximal rib bed. The transverse process may be removed as needed. A straight posterolateral or transpedicular

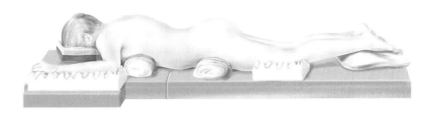

FIGURE 10–1A

POSTEROLATERAL DISK EXCISION. The patient is positioned prone, with the chest and pelvis supported on rolls.

approach may be used for more central disk pathology. A posterior approach should not be used for disk herniations that extend across the midline.

For a posterolateral approach, a straight or curvilinear incision is made 5 to 6 cm from the midline (Fig. 10–1B). Muscles are divided in layers and the rib is identified. The exposure is entirely extrapleural. Dissection is carried medially to expose the transverse process of the appropriate level. With an elevator, the rib is encircled and the neurovascular bundle is protected. The medial aspect of the rib, down to the mamillary process, is removed with the transverse process as needed (Fig. 10–1C). This permits access to the lateral aspect of the disk space. Headlight illumination and loupe magnification are helpful. Rotation of the table toward the patient's contralateral side also may facilitate visualization. The cord should not be retracted. The disk is excised

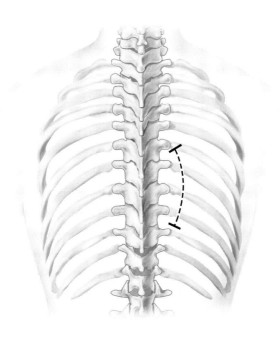

FIGURE 10–1B

A curvilinear incision is made 5 to 6 cm from the midline, with the lateral apex of the incision centered over the appropriate disk level.

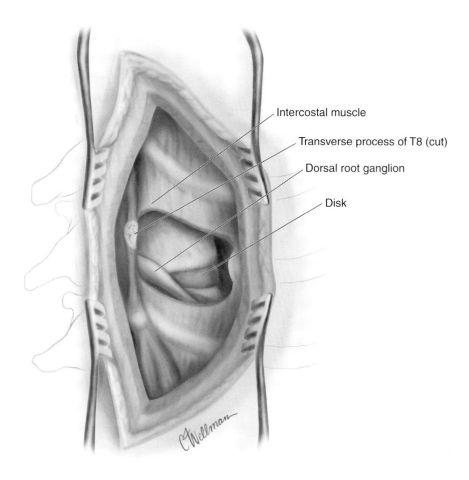

Intercostal muscle

Transverse process of T8 (cut)

Dorsal root ganglion

Disk

FIGURE 10-1C

Muscles are divided in layers and the rib is identified. Dissection is carried medially to expose the transverse process at the appropriate level. The medial aspect of the rib and the transverse process are removed. The exposure is extrapleural.

with curettes and pituitary forceps (Fig. 10–1D). Material ventral to the cord should be pushed back into the interspace and then retrieved. If the pleura are violated, a thoracostomy tube should be placed. The wound is then closed. Fusion is not necessary.

In a transpedicular approach, a midline incision is made. Self-retaining retractors are inserted and dissection is carried down to the fascia, which is split lateral to the midline. The transverse process may be resected and the pedicle visualized. The intercostal nerve root is reflected inferiorly. The pedicle is then removed with a high-speed burr. The disk is immediately inferior to the pedicle; once the pedicle has been removed, disk tissue can be visualized and excised. The wound is then closed over a suction drain.

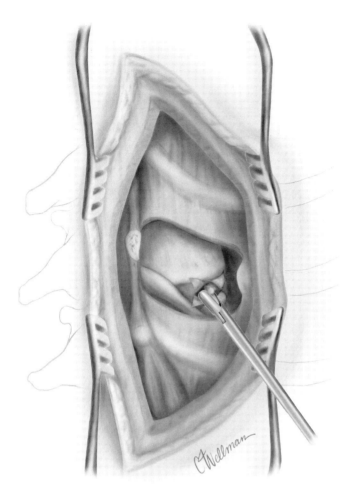

FIGURE 10-1D

The disk is excised. The cord should not be retracted. Fusion is not necessary.

POSTOPERATIVE CARE

The patient is mobilized as soon as possible postoperatively. A postoperative orthosis is not necessary.

OUTCOMES

Eighty-five percent of patients will have major pain reduction. Neurologic improvement is expected in 70% of patients. The degree of residual deficit is directly related to the degree of preoperative impairment.

COMPLICATIONS

The most common complication of posterior approach is pneumothorax. It must be recognized intraoperatively so that a thoracostomy tube can be placed. Dural tears associated with those approaches might be difficult to repair. If segmental nerves are injured, chest wall numbness can result. Retraction of the spinal cord is unnecessary and inappropriate and can result in neurologic compromise.

• ANTERIOR DISK EXCISION

SUMMARY

Anterior transthoracic disk excision of a herniated thoracic disk is indicated for myelopathy due to midline disk herniation. The disk is often calcified and not amenable to a posterolateral approach. Recently, thoracoscopic procedures have been described with the hope that the morbidity will be less, due to the limited exposure.

For the isolated disk herniation, the most common location is central or central–lateral, accounting for 60% to 80%. The most commonly involved level is T_{11-12}. Three-fourths of herniations occur in the lower thoracic spine, between T_8 and T_{11}.

PRESENTATION

Patients with midline thoracic disk herniations have myelopathic symptoms. Pain in the trunk region and the lower extremities is present. Spasticity, sensory deficits, and difficulty with ambulation occur. Clonus, hyperreflexia, and diffuse weakness are found on examination. Up to one-third of patients will have GU or GI dysfunction.

NONOPERATIVE CARE

A brief period of rest, anti-inflammatory medications, and analgesics may be indicated. The use of an orthosis is controversial. The efficacy of physical therapy has not been proven. Oral and epidural steroid therapy has not been proven to be effective in that region. When frank myelopathic symptoms are present, the treatment is surgical.

DIAGNOSTIC STUDIES

Plain radiographs might show calcification of the posterior aspects of the annulus fibrosus and the overall alignment of the spine. Patients with more kyphosis of the spine are more prone to neurologic problems with thoracic disk herniations. Instability is uncommon. MRI is the imaging procedure of choice and should show the extent of the herniation, any abnormalities related to cord compression, or parenchymal changes within the spinal cord. Myelogram with CT also might be useful but has generally been supplanted by MRI.

PROCEDURE

ANTERIOR DISK EXCISION (FIG. 10–2)

POSITIONING

Double lumen intubation is useful because it permits deflation of the lung. The patient is placed in a true lateral position (Fig. 10–2A). The operative level is determined by palpation of the ribs and radiographic confirmation. The spine is usually approached from the left side, which avoids manipulation of the vena cava.

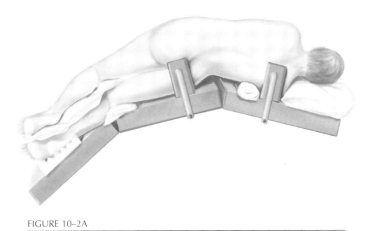

FIGURE 10–2A

ANTERIOR DISK EXCISION. The patient is placed in a true lateral decubitus position, usually left-side up. The bony prominences are well padded.

TECHNIQUE

The incision is made directly over the rib of the involved level (e.g., fifth rib for T_{5-6} disk herniation; Fig. 10–2B). In younger individuals, access may be gained through the rib interspace. In older individuals, it may be necessary to resect the rib due to inflexibility of the thoracic cage. Muscle layers are split and self-retaining retractors are inserted. The rib periosteum is elevated, taking care to protect the neurovascular bundle, and the resection is carried posteriorly to the head of the rib.

The lung is deflated and protected. The parietal pleura is incised. It is not necessary to resect segmental vessels because they lie in the mid-portion of the vertebral bodies (Fig. 10–2C). Resection of a portion of the inferior pedicle might be necessary to facilitate access to the disk space. A marker is placed in the disk space and a radiograph is obtained to confirm the appropriate level. The disk is incised and then excised with pituitary forceps (Fig. 10–2D). The posterior longitudinal ligament is visualized and excised, in addition to the posterior annulus, herniated disk, and

FIGURE 10–2B

The incision is made directly over the rib of the involved level.

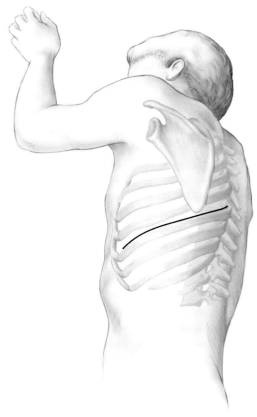

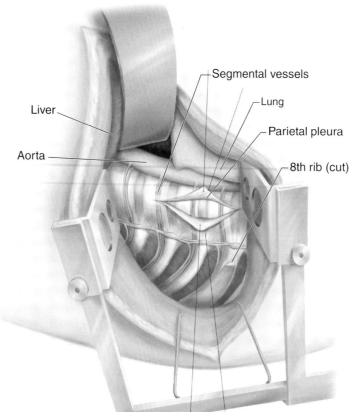

Liver

Aorta

Segmental vessels

Lung

Parietal pleura

8th rib (cut)

FIGURE 10-2C

Muscle layers are split and retractors are inserted. The neurovascular bundle is protected and the rib is resected posteriorly to its head. The lung is deflated and the pleura incised. Resection of a portion of the inferior pedicle may be necessary to facilitate access to the disk space.

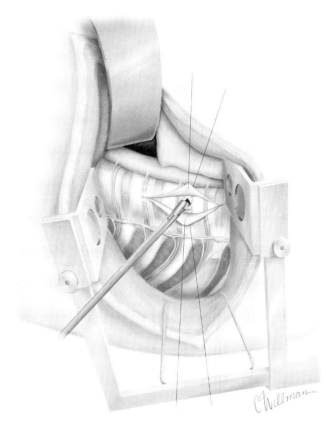

FIGURE 10-2D

After radiographic confirmation of the level, the disk is incised and excised. The posterior longitudinal ligament is visualized. Fusion is optional.

osteophytes. Although fusion is not always necessary, some surgeons, at the very least, place a morcellized portion of the rib in the interspace. A thoracostomy tube is placed and the wound is closed.

POSTOPERATIVE CARE

A postoperative radiograph of the chest is obtained to assess lung inflation. The thoracostomy tube is removed within a few days if drainage is minimal and the lung remains inflated. Postoperative pulmonary care in the form of incentive spirometry and encouragement of vigorous coughing and deep breathing are essential to facilitate complete re-expansion of the lung and prevent postoperative pneumonia. An orthosis is not required.

OUTCOMES

Eighty-five percent of patients will have major pain reduction. Neurologic improvement is expected in 70%. The degree of residual deficit is directly related to the degree of preoperative impairment.

COMPLICATIONS

Pneumothorax is part of the procedure because air is introduced into the thoracic cage. Chest tube drainage is mandatory. Neurologic deterioration is rare because of the direct approach to the cord. Thoracic or intercostal pain persists in approximately 20% of patients due to the degenerative process and the bony sequelae of the procedure.

11

SCOLIOSIS

- ## POSTERIOR FUSION WITH INSTRUMENTATION
- ## ANTERIOR RELEASE

- ## POSTERIOR FUSION WITH INSTRUMENTATION

SUMMARY

Scoliosis is a three-dimensional deformity of the spine that appears to have a genetic predisposition. It occurs more frequently in females. Idiopathic scoliosis is the most common form, occurring in approximately 2.5% of the population. It is rarely painful. In children and adolescents, surgery is performed to correct deformity and prevent progression. In adulthood, pain is the most common surgical indication.

PRESENTATION

Adolescents present with painless cosmetic deformity. The main concern with idiopathic scoliosis is curve progression, which depends on skeletal maturity and curve magnitude at presentation. The risk of progression does not end with skeletal maturity. Patients with larger curves are at increased risk for progression after skeletal maturity. Thoracic curves are more likely to progress; lumbar curves are more likely to become painful.

NONOPERATIVE CARE

In adolescents, bracing is indicated for patients with a curve magnitude of 25 to 29 degrees if curve progression of 5 degrees or more has been documented. For patients who present with curves between 30 and 40 degrees, bracing should be initiated at the first visit. Bracing is not indicated for curve magnitudes less than 20 degrees or in patients approaching the end of growth. In the adult patient, bracing will not influence curve magnitude and is of questionable benefit for pain control. The value of exercise therapy has not been proven.

DIAGNOSTIC STUDIES

Standing plain radiographs, which include the entire thoracic and lumbar spine, are required for assessment of curve magnitude. Serial radiographs are necessary to monitor curve progression in adolescents. In situations where neurologic symptoms are present, myelography with CT is indicated to visualize canal anatomy and identify potential neurologic causes of the deformity (e.g., syringomyelia and tethered cord). MRI is rarely useful because of the multiplanar deformity. In cases of severe thoracic curves, pulmonary function studies may be indicated. When surgical treatment is elected, the appropriate fusion levels must be determined. The caudal aspect of the fusion should be in an area of lordosis. In the frontal plane, vertebrae that are both neutral and stable should determine rostral–caudal extent. A stable vertebra is defined as that which is intersected by a line drawn through the center of the sacrum. Neutral is defined as the absence of significant rotation of the vertebra.

PROCEDURE

POSTERIOR FUSION WITH INSTRUMENTATION (FIG. 11–1)

POSITIONING

The patient is placed prone on rolls or on a surgical frame that allows hip extension and maintenance of lumbar lordosis (Fig. 11–1A).

TECHNIQUE

A straight longitudinal midline incision is made (Fig. 11–1B). The dissection is carried down to the spine and self-retaining retractors are placed. The exposure should extend to the tips of the transverse processes in the thoracic spine (Fig. 11–1C). In

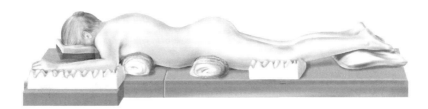

FIGURE 11–1A

POSTERIOR FUSION WITH INSTRUMENTATION. The patient is placed on rolls or a surgical frame to permit hip extension and preservation of lumbar lordosis.

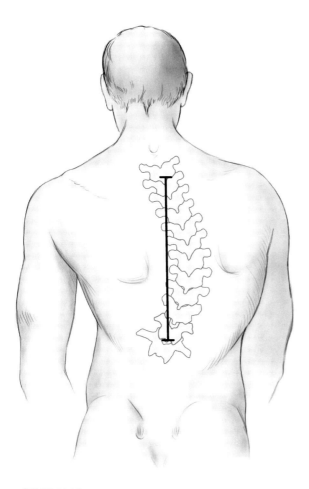

FIGURE 11–1B

A straight longitudinal, posterior midline incision is made.

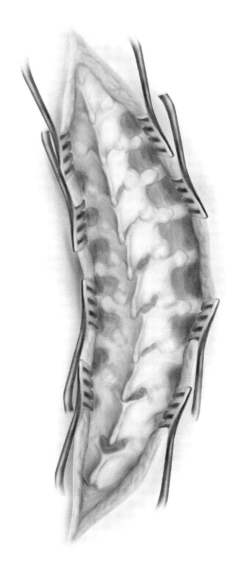

FIGURE 11-1C

Exposure should extend to the tips of the transverse processes in the thoracic spine, but can be stopped at the facets in the lumbar region.

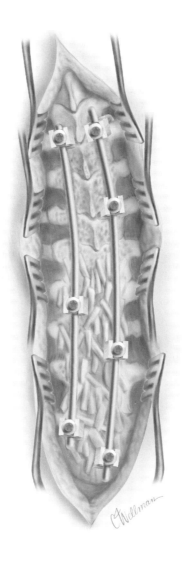

FIGURE 11-1D

End points for fusion are selected. Appropriate hook placement is determined preoperatively. Rods are bent to approximate the final desired spinal contour. Instrumentation is placed and correction is achieved. The entire posterior surface is decorticated and bone graft is applied.

the lumbar region, exposure may be stopped at the facets; if additional surface area for grafting is desired, then transverse processes are exposed.

The end points selected for fusion are identified. Spinal instrumentation is indicated in correction of deformity. Segmental systems with multiple hooks and screws are used currently because of their ability to provide segmental rotational control, correct the deformity in the frontal and sagittal planes, and restore balance. The appropriate locations of hooks and instrumentation are determined from preoperative radiographs according to curve magnitude, location, and flexibility.

Inferiorly directed hooks are generally placed over the transverse processes, and superiorly directed hooks are placed under the lamina or at the facet joint–pedicle junction. The rods are bent to approximate the final desired spinal contour. Dual parallel rods are applied to the hooks and provisionally attached, and by a combination of distraction, compression, and rotation, correction is achieved. At this stage, permanent fixation of the rods to the hooks is performed. The rods may be cross-linked, if desired.

Once instrumentation has been placed and correction achieved, the posterior surface area is decorticated with an osteotome, gouge, or high-speed burr, and morcellized iliac bone graft is applied (Fig. 11–1D).

Evoked potential monitoring and/or a wake-up test are used to make sure that no neurologic problems have occurred as a result of the surgical correction. A drain may be placed before closure.

POSTOPERATIVE CARE

With the use of segmental instrumentation systems, no postoperative orthotic immobilization is necessary.

OUTCOMES

With segmental fixation devices, correction of 50% to 80% of curve magnitude can be achieved in young individuals. In older patients with more rigid spinal deformities, less correction is indicated. The likelihood of achieving solid arthrodesis is approximately 90% in the adolescent and 80% in the adult. Postoperative pain relief in the adult is unpredictable.

COMPLICATIONS

The most feared complication is paralysis. Assessing spinal flexibility preoperatively and using appropriate neurologic monitoring techniques can minimize that risk. Other complications are failure of fusion, adjacent segment degeneration, coronal or sagittal imbalance, and iatrogenic flat back deformity. Failure of fixation is rare. Complications are more likely in older individuals or those with osteoporosis.

• ANTERIOR RELEASE

SUMMARY

Larger curves (60 degrees or greater) can be treated by anterior release followed by posterior segmental instrumentation and fusion. It can be performed as two separate surgical procedures or on the same day as a two-part operation.

PRESENTATION

Adolescents present with painless cosmetic deformity. The main concern with idiopathic scoliosis is curve progression, which depends on skeletal maturity and curve magnitude. The risk of progression does not end with skeletal maturation. Patients with larger curves are at increased risk for progression after skeletal maturity. Thoracic curves are more likely to progress; lumbar curves are more likely to become painful.

NONOPERATIVE CARE

In adolescents, bracing is indicated for patients with a curve magnitude of 25 to 29 degrees if curve progression of 5 degrees or more has been documented. For patients who present with curves between 30 and 40 degrees, bracing should be initiated at the first visit. Bracing is not indicated for curve magnitudes less than 20 degrees or in patients approaching the end of growth. In the adult patient, bracing will not influence curve magnitude and is of questionable benefit for pain control. The value of exercise therapy has not been proven.

DIAGNOSTIC STUDIES

Standing plain radiographs visualizing the entire thoracic and lumbar spine are required to assess curve magnitude. Serial radiographs are necessary to monitor curve progression in adolescents. In situations where neurologic symptoms are present, myelogram with CT is indicated to visualize canal anatomy and identify potential neurologic causes of the deformity. MRI is rarely useful because of the multiple plane deformity. In cases of severe thoracic curves, pulmonary function studies may be indicated.

PROCEDURE

ANTERIOR RELEASE (FIG. 11–2)

POSITIONING

Double lumen tube intubation is used because it allows the lung to be deflated, thereby permitting better access to the spine. The patient is placed in a lateral position on the side of curve concavity (Fig. 11–2A).

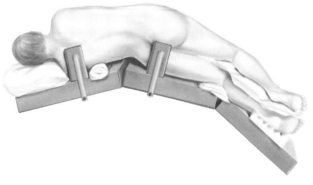

FIGURE 11–2A

ANTERIOR RELEASE. The patient is placed in a lateral position, on the side of curve concavity.

TECHNIQUE

The approach is through a rib bed with resection of the rib (Fig. 11–2B). Self-retaining retractors are placed. The periosteum is elevated from the rib and the neurovascular bundle is protected. The rib is resected and saved for use as graft.

The disks are identified and excised and the anterior longitudinal ligament is released (Fig. 11–2C). The segmental vessels usually can be preserved because of their location in the middle portion of the thoracic vertebrae. End-plates are decorticated and morcellized bone graft is placed into the debrided interspaces (Fig. 11–2D). Thoracoscopic approaches for this procedure have been described.

A thoracostomy tube is placed and the wound is closed.

After completion of the anterior release, the patient is turned prone for the posterior procedure.

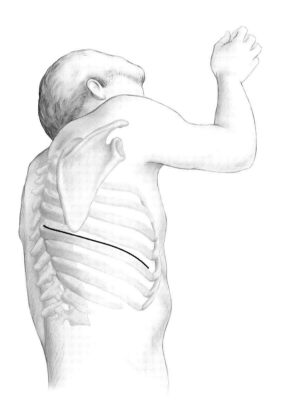

FIGURE 11–2B

The incision is made over the appropriate rib.

FIGURE 11-2C

The rib is resected after periosteal elevation and protection of the neurovascular bundle. Segmental vessels usually can be preserved. Anterior longitudinal ligament is released and disks are excised.

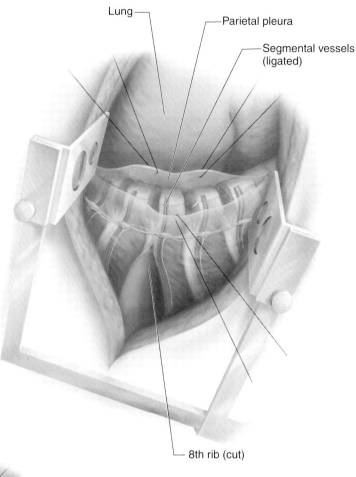

Lung

Parietal pleura

Segmental vessels (ligated)

8th rib (cut)

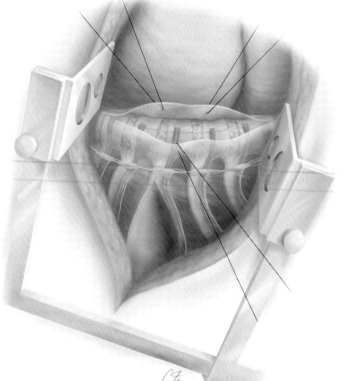

FIGURE 11-2D

After disk excision and ligament release, end-plates are decorticated and morcellized bone graft obtained from the resected rib is placed into the interspaces.

POSTOPERATIVE CARE

A postoperative radiograph of the chest is obtained to assess lung inflation. The thoracostomy tube is removed within a few days if drainage is minimal and the lung remains inflated. Postoperative pulmonary care in the form of incentive spirometry and vigorous encouragement of coughing and deep breathing are essential to facilitate complete re-expansion of the lung and prevent postoperative pneumonia. An orthosis is not required.

OUTCOMES

More correction and higher fusion rate are expected with combined anterior and posterior procedures.

COMPLICATIONS

Pneumothorax is part of the procedure because air is introduced into the thoracic cage. Chest tube drainage is mandatory. Neurologic complications are rare. Other complications are pneumonia, spine and chest wall pain, and, rarely, pseudarthrosis.

12

KYPHOSIS

- ANTERIOR RELEASE
- POSTERIOR STABILIZATION AND CORRECTION

- ANTERIOR RELEASE

SUMMARY

The most common causes of kyphosis are congenital, posttraumatic, or acquired Scheuermann's disease. Acquired kyphosis is uncommon, occurring most frequently in adolescent males. It is probably related to growth problems of the anterior vertebral bodies. Brace treatment sometimes can be effective. Surgery may be indicated when there is a cosmetic deformity (kyphosis of 70 degrees or greater) and when pulmonary function is compromised.

PRESENTATION

Congenital kyphosis can present with neurologic deficit; it is frequently progressive in the growing spine. In postfracture kyphosis, pain is the most common complaint. In Scheuermann's disease, pain is a frequent complaint, which is possibly due to posturally induced muscle fatigue. Pulmonary function is rarely compromised.

NONOPERATIVE CARE

Nonsteroidal anti-inflammatory medications, analgesics, and physical therapy may be useful for symptomatic relief. In adolescent kyphosis, bracing may be used to decrease mechanical forces on the anterior aspect of the growing spine.

DIAGNOSTIC STUDIES

The etiology and extent of the deformity are apparent on plain films. MRI or myelogram CT is indicated, particularly in cases of congenital kyphosis, to rule out underlying neurologic abnormalities.

111

PROCEDURE

ANTERIOR RELEASE (FIG. 12–1)

POSITIONING

Double lumen tube intubation can be used to allow the lung to be deflated, thereby permitting better access to the spine. The patient is placed in lateral position, usually on the right side (Fig. 12–1A).

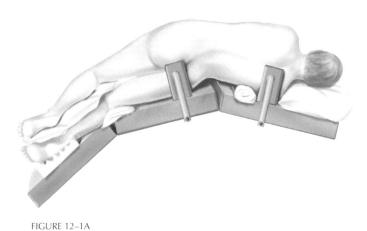

FIGURE 12–1A

KYPHOSIS—ANTERIOR RELEASE. The patient is placed in a lateral decubitus position, left side up. The bony prominences are padded.

TECHNIQUE

The incision is made over the rib at the apex of the kyphosis (Fig. 12–1B). The periosteum is stripped, the neurovascular bundle is protected, and the rib is resected.

Anterior release is performed over the extent of the kyphosis. Release of the anterior longitudinal ligament and disk excision to the posterior annulus is performed (Fig. 12–1C). Morcellized bone graft may be placed in the disk spaces (Fig. 12–1D). Segmental vessels are preserved where possible.

The resected rib is morcellized and placed into the debrided interspaces after decortication of the end-plates.

A thoracostomy tube is then placed and the wound is closed. The anterior procedure is followed by posterior segmental instrumentation correction. The risk of neurologic injury is greatest during the posterior correction. The use of evoked potential monitoring and/or a wake-up test minimizes that risk.

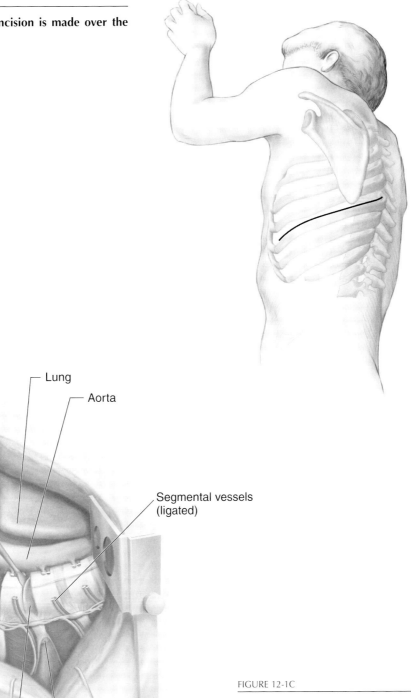

FIGURE 12–1B

A curvilinear incision is made over the apical rib.

Lung

Aorta

Segmental vessels
(ligated)

Vertebral end-plate

8th rib (cut)

FIGURE 12-1C

After rib resection and division of thoracic musculature, the thoracic cavity is entered and the lung is retracted. The pleura is incised two segments proximal and two segments distal to the apex of the deformity. Segmental vessels are ligated as necessary.

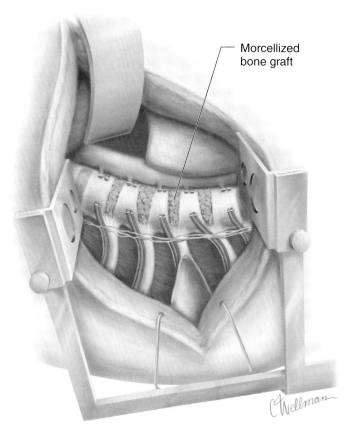

Morcellized
bone graft

FIGURE 12-1D

End-plates are decorticated. The resected rib is morcellized and placed into the appropriate interspaces.

POSTOPERATIVE CARE

The patient is mobilized as soon as possible postoperatively. A postoperative orthosis is not necessary.

OUTCOMES

Combined anterior and posterior procedures for kyphosis result in better correction and a higher fusion rate than posterior procedures alone. Deformity correction of approximately 50% is expected.

COMPLICATIONS

Complications from anterior release include injury to the great vessels or spinal cord. These are minimized by meticulous surgical approach. The risk of neurologic complication is highest during attempted correction of severe congenital kyphotic deformity. Breathing difficulties and pneumonia related to the approach can occur in addition to spinal cord injury and chest wall pain.

• POSTERIOR STABILIZATION AND CORRECTION

SUMMARY

The most common causes of kyphosis are congenital, posttraumatic, or acquired Scheuermann's disease. Acquired kyphosis is uncommon, occurring most frequently in adolescent males. It is probably related to growth problems of the anterior vertebral bodies. Brace treatment sometimes can be effective. Surgery may be indicated when there is a cosmetic deformity (kyphosis of 70 degrees or greater) and when pulmonary function is compromised.

Posterior stabilization and correction of kyphotic deformity are indicated for moderate kyphosis (60 to 80 degrees).

PRESENTATION

Congenital kyphosis can present with neurologic deficit; it is frequently progressive in the growing spine. In postfracture kyphosis, pain is the most common complaint. In Scheuermann's disease, pain is a frequent complaint, which is possibly due to posturally induced muscle fatigue. Pulmonary function is rarely compromised.

NONOPERATIVE CARE

Nonsteroidal anti-inflammatory medications, analgesics, and physical therapy may be useful for symptomatic relief. In adolescent kyphosis, bracing may be used to decrease mechanical forces on the anterior aspect of the growing spine.

DIAGNOSTIC STUDIES

The etiology and extent of the deformity are apparent on plain films. MRI or myelogram CT is indicated, particularly in cases of congenital kyphosis, to rule out underlying neurologic abnormalities.

PROCEDURE

POSTERIOR STABILIZATION AND CORRECTION (FIG. 12–2)

POSITIONING

The patient is positioned prone on rolls or in a surgical frame that provides for extension of the hips (Fig. 12–2A).

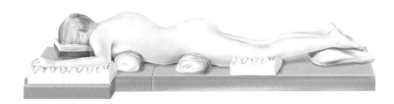

FIGURE 12–2A

**KYPHOSIS—POSTERIOR STABILIZATION AND CORREC-
TION. The patient is positioned prone, with the hips extended.**

To minimize the risk of neurologic complications after deformity correction, evoked potential monitoring and/or wake-up test are indicated.

An incision is made in the midline and dissection is carried down to the spine (Fig. 12–2B). Lateral exposure should extend to the tips of the transverse processes. Self-retaining retractors are inserted (Fig. 12–2C).

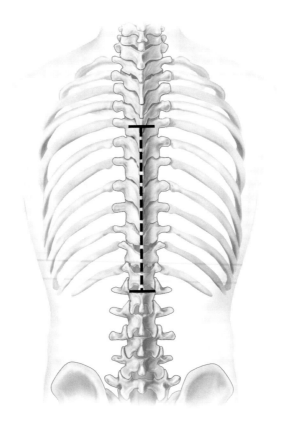

FIGURE 12–2B

The skin is incised in the midline centered over the apex of the kyphosis.

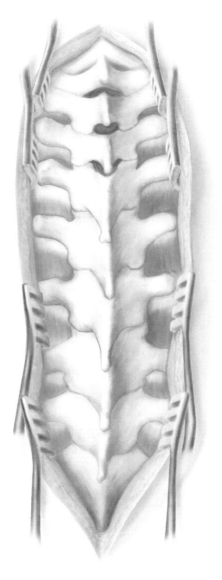

FIGURE 12-2C

The spine is exposed in a standard posterior manner to the tips of the transverse processes.

Segmental instrumentation using multiple hooks and parallel rods is performed and a gradual correction force is applied in a compression mode. Superiorly directed hooks are placed under the lamina or in the facet joint–pedicle junction. Inferiorly directed hooks usually are placed over the transverse process or under the lamina. When the desired correction is achieved, the rods are permanently affixed to the hooks. Morcellized bone graft is placed over the decorticated posterior elements. The rods may be connected by cross-linking (Fig. 12–2D).

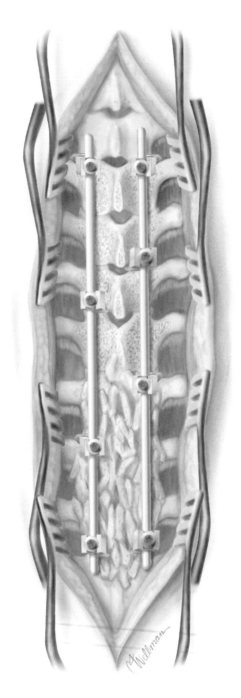

FIGURE 12-2D

Segmental instrumentation is performed. Gradual correction forces are applied in a compressive mode. Morcellized graft is placed over the decorticated posterior elements.

POSTOPERATIVE CARE

With posterior segmental fixation, postoperative orthotic immobilization is optional.

OUTCOMES

Fifty-percent correction in curve magnitude in the sagittal plane is expected. Muscle fatigue due to the kyphosis is usually improved. Failure of fusion occurs in approximately 15% of cases.

COMPLICATIONS

Neurologic injury is rare but can occur. It can be related to hook placement or attempts at excessive correction. In thin patients, local pain due to prominent instrumentation can occur. Failure of fixation is rare.

13

FRACTURES

- POSTERIOR REDUCTION AND STABILIZATION
- ANTERIOR REDUCTION AND STABILIZATION

- POSTERIOR REDUCTION AND STABILIZATION

SUMMARY

Spinal injuries occur most frequently in young adult males. Noncontiguous spine fractures can occur in up to 20% of those with spine fractures. Fractures of the thoracic and lumbar spine are divided into four categories. **Compression fractures** involve the anterior vertebral column. These are stable unless more than 50% of vertebral height is lost or they occur over multiple levels. **Burst fractures** are uncommon in the thoracic spine because of the anatomic kyphosis of this region, which minimizes loading of the middle column. **Fracture–dislocations** are relatively common in this region and are the result of high-energy trauma. Neurologic injury is common in fracture–dislocations. **Flexion–distraction injuries** are the result of ligament or bone disruption, which is initiated posteriorly. Surgical treatment is indicated for instability and neurologic injury. In the thoracic spine, surgery is performed most frequently for fracture–dislocations.

PRESENTATION

Most of these injuries are the result of motor vehicle accidents. Thoracic pain is present and a kyphotic deformity may be evident. Neurologic injury is most common in fracture–dislocations. At the thoracic level, the spinal cord is vulnerable and traumatic instability often results in incomplete or complete paralysis. A complete trauma and neurologic assessment is mandatory.

121

NONOPERATIVE CARE

Stable fractures can be managed with an orthosis. These fractures include most compression fractures and the stable burst fractures.

DIAGNOSTIC STUDIES

Plain radiographs will show the type of injury and alignment of the thoracic spine. The test of choice to determine the extent of bony injury and canal compromise is CT. MRI is useful to assess soft tissue injury and the status of the neural elements.

PROCEDURE

POSTERIOR REDUCTION AND STABILIZATION (FIG. 13–1)

POSITIONING

The patient is placed in a prone position with transverse rolls across the superior aspect of the thorax and pelvis (Fig. 13–1A). The position permits gentle reduction of the kyphosis.

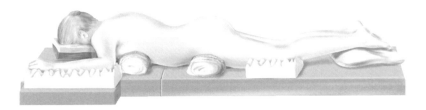

FIGURE 13–1A

FRACTURES—POSTERIOR REDUCTION AND STABILIZATION. The patient is placed in the prone position with rolls to reduce the kyphosis.

TECHNIQUE

A midline incision is made over the injury (Fig. 13–1B). A standard posterior exposure is performed (Fig. 13–1C). Instrumentation is employed with two segments fixated above and two segments below. Claw-type fixation is indicated, with inferiorly facing hooks placed over the transverse processes or lamina and the superiorly facing hooks beneath the lamina or at the facet joint–pedicle junction. The claw configuration is applied above and below the fracture–dislocation site. The rod is contoured to correct the kyphotic deformity on insertion. Rods are locked in place.

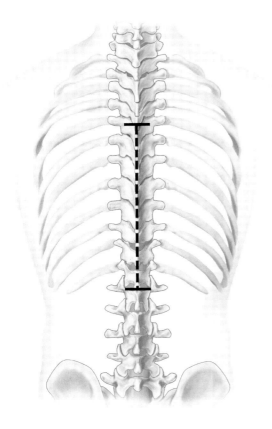

FIGURE 13–1B

A midline incision is made over the level of the fracture from at least two levels above to two levels below.

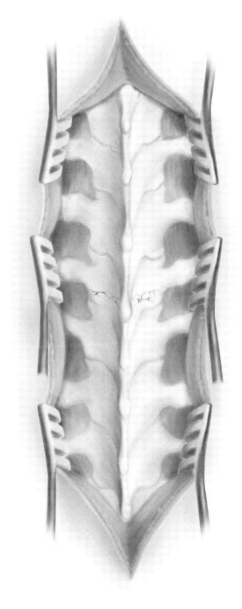

FIGURE 13-1C

The fascia is split in the midline and lateral dissection is extended to the tips of the transverse processes. Care is taken during muscle stripping of the fracture level.

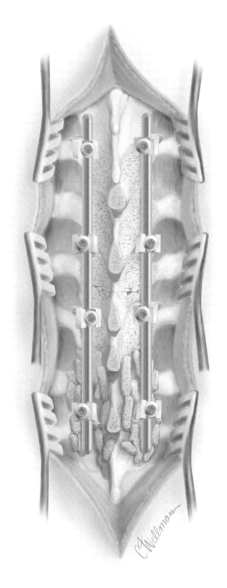

FIGURE 13-1D

A claw configuration is placed above and below the fracture. The rods are contoured to correct the kyphosis. After hardware placement, posterior elements are decorticated and bone graft is placed.

The decorticated posterior elements are covered with morcellized iliac crest bone graft (Fig. 13–1D).

The wound is closed over a suction drain.

POSTOPERATIVE CARE

The use of orthotic support is optional depending on the nature of the injury and the stability of fixation. Patients with neurologic injury are enrolled in a rehabilitation program.

OUTCOMES

Functional outcome depends on the residual neurologic impairment. Instrumentation problems are uncommon, but can occur, with the use of segmental fixation. Failure of fusion is rare in traumatic injuries.

Rehabilitation may be hampered in patients with multiple injuries.

COMPLICATIONS

Infection is rare, as are complications related to intraoperative neurologic injury or dural tear.

• ANTERIOR REDUCTION AND STABILIZATION

SUMMARY

Anterior reduction and stabilization are indicated for fractures of the thoracic spine that involve the anterior and middle columns. Such fractures most commonly affect the inferior regions of the thoracic spine adjacent to the thoracolumbar junction. Anterior procedures are indicated when bone from the middle column (posterior aspect of the vertebral body) intrudes into the spinal canal. A direct anterior approach permits spinal canal decompression and stabilization.

PRESENTATION

These fractures are generally of a high-energy nature and most commonly related to motor vehicle accidents. Back pain is a predominant feature and neurologic injury may be present. At the thoracic level, the spinal cord is vulnerable and traumatic instability often results in incomplete or complete paralysis. A complete trauma and neurologic assessment is mandatory.

NONOPERATIVE CARE

Stable fractures may be managed with an orthosis. These fractures include most compression fractures and stable burst fractures. The most important decision is which surgical approach to use, anterior or posterior.

DIAGNOSTIC STUDIES

Plain radiographs suggest the mechanism of injury and allow for classification. CT shows the extent of osseous comminution and canal compromise. MRI shows the status of the neurologic and soft tissue structures. Myelogram CT is an alternative imaging procedure that is used rarely.

PROCEDURE

ANTERIOR REDUCTION AND STABILIZATION (FIG. 13–2)

POSITIONING

The patient is placed in a lateral position, on the right side (Fig. 13–2A).

TECHNIQUE

An oblique incision is made over the rib at the level of the fracture (Fig. 13–2B). The rib is excised, usually subperiosteally, to the rib head. Neurovascular structures are protected. The rib may be preserved in younger individuals with a flexible thoracic

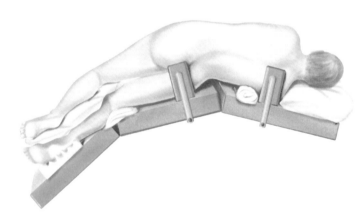

FIGURE 13–2A

FRACTURES—ANTERIOR REDUCTION AND STABILIZATION. Positioning.

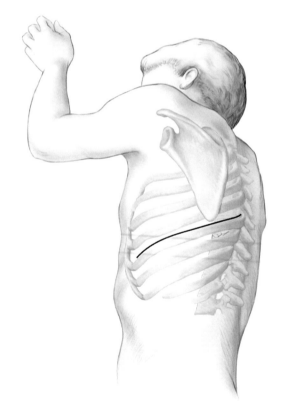

FIGURE 13–2B

A curvilinear incision is made over the apical rib.

cage. Radiographic confirmation of the involved segment is obtained. Segmental vessels at the level involved are ligated and retracted (Fig. 13–2C). The comminuted vertebral body elements and adjacent disks are resected. The epidural space is thoroughly decompressed (Fig. 13–2D). After manual reduction of the kyphosis, a tricortical strut graft is placed between the adjacent intact vertebral bodies and a plate-screw device is fixed to the spine (Fig. 13–2E). Most devices allow for some compression to aid in healing. A thoracostomy tube is placed before closure.

FIGURE 13-2C

After rib resection and division of thoracic musculature, the thoracic cavity is entered and the lung is retracted. The pleura is incised one segment proximal and one segment distal to the fracture. Segmental vessels are ligated.

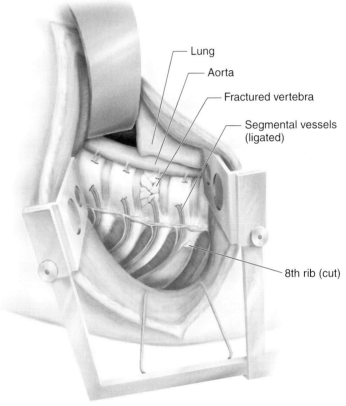

Lung

Aorta

Fractured vertebra

Segmental vessels (ligated)

8th rib (cut)

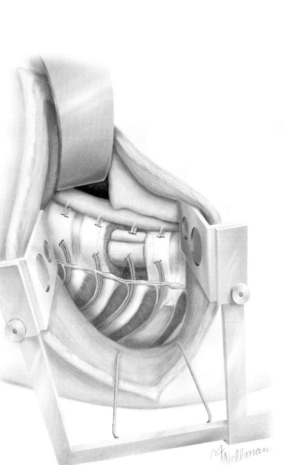

FIGURE 13-2D

Comminuted vertebral body elements and adjacent disks are resected and decompression is performed. The kyphosis can be reduced manually.

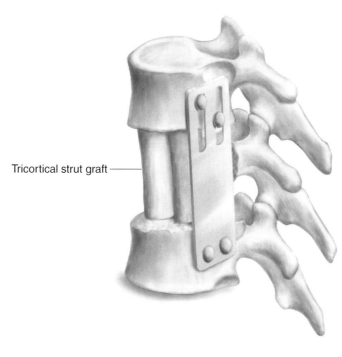

Tricortical strut graft

FIGURE 13-2E

Rostral and caudal end-plates are prepared and a structural graft is placed. Anterior fixation can be used.

POSTOPERATIVE CARE

Immobilization in a thoracolumbar orthosis is recommended. A rehabilitation program can assist in obtaining maximal function particularly in those individuals with residual neurologic impairment.

A postoperative radiograph of the chest is obtained to assess lung inflation. The thoracostomy tube is removed within a few days, if drainage is minimal and the lung remains inflated. Postoperative pulmonary care in the form of incentive spirometry and vigorous encouragement of coughing and deep breathing are essential to facilitate complete re-expansion of the lung and prevent postoperative pneumonia.

OUTCOMES

Neurologic improvement may be expected in incomplete injuries regardless of the treatment method. True complete lesions rarely demonstrate neurologic improvement. Correction of the kyphosis and solid arthrodesis is anticipated. Major residual back pain is uncommon after this procedure.

COMPLICATIONS

Most complications relate to the thoracotomy. Pneumothorax can occur, and other pulmonary complications such as pneumonia are seen. Loss of fixation is rare and when it occurs can be treated by re-operation or supplementary posterior fixation.

Complications from anterior fusion also include injury to the great vessels or spinal cord. These are minimized by meticulous surgical approach. The risk of neurologic complication is highest during attempted correction of kyphotic deformity. Breathing difficulties and pneumonia related to the approach can occur, as can spinal cord and chest wall pain.

14

TUMORS

- POSTERIOR DECOMPRESSION
  AND STABILIZATION
  OF THORACIC TUMOR

- ANTERIOR CORPECTOMY
  AND STABILIZATION
  OF THORACIC TUMOR WITH
  POLYMETHYLMETHACRYLATE

- POSTERIOR DECOMPRESSION AND
  STABILIZATION OF THORACIC TUMOR

SUMMARY

Most tumors affecting the thoracic spine are metastatic. Surgery is indicated with severe or progressive deformity or neurologic compromise. The decision to approach a tumor posteriorly must be made with caution because most metastatic lesions involve the vertebral body; thus, surgical care is directed predominantly anteriorly. Posterior procedures are indicated when the lesion is of a unilateral nature and access can be gained through a posterolateral approach. Life expectancy also should be considered when a decision is made concerning surgical treatment.

PRESENTATION

Back pain and neurologic dysfunction are the usual presenting symptoms of tumors within the thoracic region. Due to the anatomy of the thoracic spine, neurologic dysfunction is more likely with tumors in this region than in other areas of the spine. History of a primary tumor elsewhere may exist, but in 10% of patients, a metastatic thoracic lesion may be the initial presentation. This is more likely in individuals older than 45 years.

131

NONOPERATIVE CARE

Tumors that are radiosensitive and do not involve more than 50% of the vertebral body can be treated with radiation therapy and brace immobilization. Tumors meeting operative criteria are those causing neurologic dysfunction or structural compromise.

DIAGNOSTIC STUDIES

Plain films are indicated to assess spinal alignment and estimate the extent of osseous destruction. CT is the test of choice for delineating bony destruction; MRI shows the extent of the tumor and the status of structural compromise.

PROCEDURE

POSTERIOR DECOMPRESSION AND STABILIZATION OF THORACIC TUMOR (FIG. 14–1)

POSITIONING

The procedure is performed typically with the patient in the prone position, although lateral approaches have been described. Transverse rolls are placed beneath the thorax and pelvis (Fig. 14–1A).

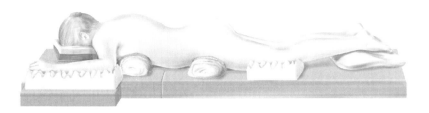

FIGURE 14–1A

TUMORS—POSTERIOR DECOMPRESSION AND STABILIZATION OF THORACIC TUMOR. The patient is positioned prone.

TECHNIQUE

A midline incision is made over the level of the tumor (Fig. 14–1B). Paraspinous muscles are carefully dissected out to the level of the proximal rib. Decompression is performed through a transpedicular approach. If anterior bone grafting is desired, a more extensive lateral approach (costotransversectomy) may be used, with excision of the proximal portion of one or two ribs. Segmental neurovascular bundles are preserved. It is important to keep the exposure extrapleural.

The spinal canal is decompressed by the removal of bone and tumor with rongeurs and curettes (Fig. 14–1C). A transpedicular or costotransversectomy approach provides unilateral decompression. A bilateral approach will permit a more

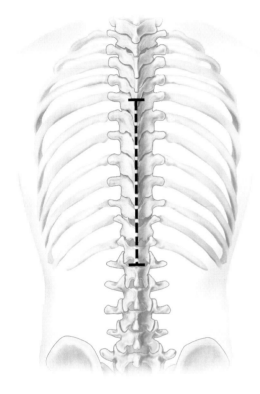

FIGURE 14–1B

The incision is made in the midline two levels above to two levels below the affected segment.

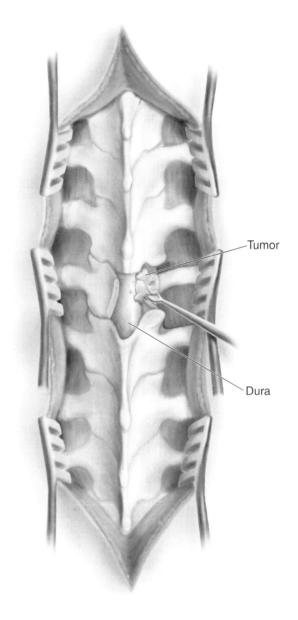

FIGURE 14-1C

The fascia is split in the midline and exposure is carried laterally to the tips of the transverse processes. Care must be taken with exposure of the involved level because of suboptimal bone quality and the risk of neurologic injury. After exposure, transpedicular decompression is performed. The cord must not be retracted.

thorough decompression; this is uncommon, however, because more extensive tumors are usually managed through an anterior approach. After decompression, bone graft (iliac crest or rib or structural allograft) is inserted. Posterior segmental instrumentation with a hook–rod construct is then applied. A two-segment claw configuration is used superiorly. Inferiorly, a double-level claw configuration is used in the thoracic spine (Fig. 14–1D). In the lumbar spine, pedicle screw devices may be substituted. Supplementary bone grafting is performed over decorticated posterior elements. The wound is then closed over suction drains.

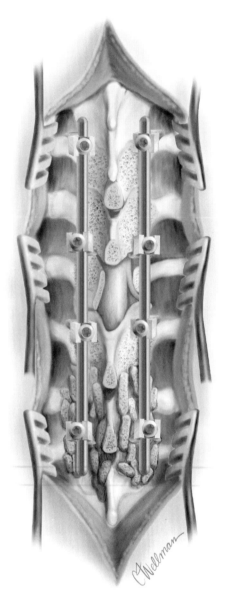

FIGURE 14-1D

After decompression, posterior segmental instrumentation is applied with a two-segment claw construct rostral and caudal to the involved level. The spinal cord is protected, the posterior elements are decorticated, and bone graft is applied.

POSTOPERATIVE CARE

A chest x-ray is essential to assess inflation of the lung. A thoracolumbar orthosis is generally used. When neurologic compromise is present, a rehabilitation program is indicated. Supplemental radiation therapy and chemotherapy may be indicated, depending on the type of neoplasm. If possible, radiotherapy should be delayed for 3 weeks to minimize wound complications.

OUTCOMES

Back pain and neurologic compromise are expected to improve postoperatively. Long-term prognosis depends on the nature of the tumor and its responsiveness to surgical and adjunctive therapy. The median survival time for individuals presenting with metastatic lesions of the spine is 2 years.

COMPLICATIONS

There is a risk of pneumothorax with costotransversectomy. Displacement of the anteriorly placed bone graft can occur. Posterior segmental instrumentation problems are uncommon but can occur depending on bone quality. Inadequate decompression is more likely to occur with a posterior than with an anterior approach. The nature of the disease and the use of adjunctive therapy may predispose individuals to healing problems and infection.

• ANTERIOR CORPECTOMY AND STABILIZATION OF THORACIC TUMOR WITH POLYMETHYLMETHACRYLATE

SUMMARY

Most tumors affecting the thoracic spine are metastatic. Surgery is indicated with severe or progressive deformity or neurologic compromise. The treatment of an extensive tumor involving the vertebral body is similar to the treatment of fractures in this area. A thoracotomy approach permits the best access to the tumor. Complete resection of the tumor often is not feasible. For individuals with a life expectancy of less than 6 months, synthetic polymethylmethacrylate rather than bone graft can be used for structural support. Due to the probability of loosening, polymethylmethacrylate should not be used in patients with a longer life expectancy. Supplemental internal fixation is optional.

PRESENTATION

Back pain and neurologic dysfunction are the usual presenting symptoms of tumors within the thoracic region. Due to the anatomy of the thoracic spine, neurologic dysfunction is more likely with tumors in this region than in other areas of the spine. In

10% of patients, a metastatic thoracic lesion may be the initial presentation. This is more likely in individuals older than 45 years.

NONOPERATIVE CARE

Tumors that are radiosensitive and do not involve more than 50% of the vertebral body can be treated with radiation therapy and brace immobilization. Tumors meeting operative criteria are those causing neurologic dysfunction or structural compromise.

DIAGNOSTIC STUDIES

Plain films are indicated to assess spinal alignment and estimate the extent of osseous destruction. CT is the test of choice for delineating bony destruction; MRI shows the extent of the tumor and the status of structural compromise.

PROCEDURE

ANTERIOR CORPECTOMY AND STABILIZATION OF THORACIC TUMOR WITH POLYMETHYLMETHACRYLATE (FIG. 14–2)

POSITIONING

Double lumen intubation can be used to permit deflation of the lung and improve surgical access. The patient is placed in true lateral position (Fig. 14–2A).

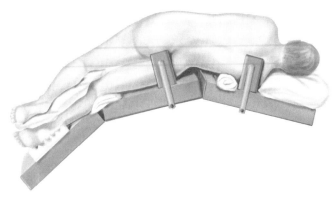

FIGURE 14–2A

TUMORS—ANTERIOR CORPECTOMY AND STABILIZATION OF THORACIC TUMOR WITH POLYMETHYLMETHACRYLATE (PMMA). The patient is placed in a true lateral decubitus position, with the shoulders perpendicular to the floor.

TECHNIQUE

Access is gained through the rib bed of the rib superior to the level involved (Fig. 14–2B). During rib resection, the neurovascular bundle should be protected. The thoracic cavity is entered through the pleura and the lesion is identified and confirmed with radiographic control (Fig. 14–2C). Segmental vessels are ligated as appropriate. The tumor is excised with rongeurs and curettes. Spinal canal decompression is performed as indicated. Resection of the tumor is carried to healthy-appearing, bleeding, cancellous bone. Reduction of kyphosis is achieved by manual pressure on the posterior aspect of the spine at the level involved. Methylmethacrylate is prepared and molded into a cylindrical configuration and inserted into the defect (Fig. 14–2D). Supplementary plate-screw fixation also can be used. A thoracostomy tube is placed and the wound is closed.

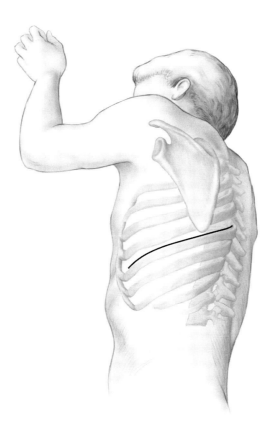

FIGURE 14–2B

An incision is made parallel to the rib bed immediately superior to the involved level.

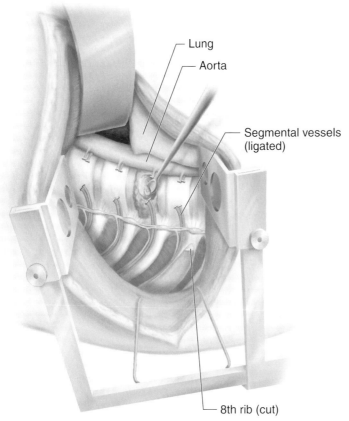

Lung

Aorta

Segmental vessels (ligated)

8th rib (cut)

FIGURE 14-2C

The rib is resected and the lung is deflated. The thoracic cavity is entered through the pleura. The lesion is identified. Segmental vessels are ligated.

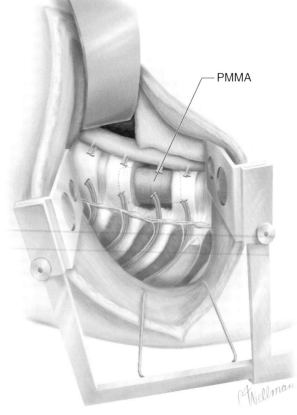

PMMA

FIGURE 14-2D

The tumor is excised *in toto* along with the rostral and caudal disks. After reduction of the kyphosis, a cylinder of PMMA is inserted into the defect.

POSTOPERATIVE CARE

A chest x-ray is essential to assess inflation of the lung. The chest tube is removed when postoperative drainage is minimal. A thoracolumbar orthosis is generally employed. When neurologic compromise is present, a rehabilitation program is indicated. Supplemental radiation therapy and chemotherapy may be indicated, depending on the type of neoplasm. If possible, radiotherapy should be delayed for 3 weeks to minimize wound complications.

COMPLICATIONS

Pneumothorax is part of the procedure. Loss of fixation or stability is uncommon with polymethylmethacrylate. Wound healing problems and infection are more common in patients undergoing radiation therapy and chemotherapy.

15

INFECTION

- ## DRAINAGE OF EPIDURAL ABSCESS
- ## CORPECTOMY AND INTERBODY FUSION

- ## DRAINAGE OF EPIDURAL ABSCESS

SUMMARY

Epidural abscess causing neurologic compromise is rare in the thoracic region. It is seen most commonly in immunocompromised patients, particularly those with diabetes mellitus.

PRESENTATION

Initial presenting symptoms can be vague. Low-grade fever and constitutional symptoms can occur. The diagnosis usually is suggested by progressive neurologic deterioration localized to a thoracic level. An abscess causing neurologic compromise is an indication for urgent surgical drainage.

NONOPERATIVE CARE

A minor neurologic deficit that is not functionally debilitating can, on occasion, be treated with intravenous antibiotics, immobilization, and observation. Most patients, however, present with serious neurologic dysfunction and emergent surgical care is indicated.

DIAGNOSTIC STUDIES

Plain radiographs assess overall alignment of the spine and demonstrate osseous destruction. Radionuclide scans may show vertebral osteomyelitis or other sites of involvement in the skeleton. MRI, however, is the study of choice because it shows the extent of the abscess and the status of the neurologic tissues.

PROCEDURE

DRAINAGE OF EPIDURAL ABSCESS (FIG. 15–1)

POSITIONING

The patient is placed in a prone position (Fig. 15–1A).

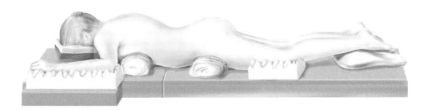

FIGURE 15–1A

INFECTION—DRAINAGE OF EPIDURAL ABSCESS. The patient is positioned prone.

TECHNIQUE

An incision is made in the midline and a traditional laminectomy approach is performed (Fig. 15–1B). Posterior elements are excised with the use of Kerrison rongeurs.

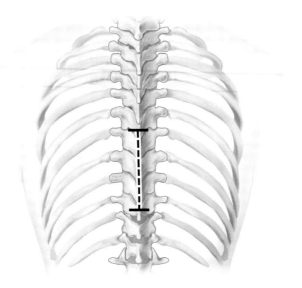

FIGURE 15–1B

An incision is made in the midline over the involved level.

On entry into the epidural space, gross purulence or a gelatinous substance might be encountered (Fig. 15–1C). This material is gently debrided throughout its extent. Antibiotic irrigation is used. Stabilization is generally not necessary unless vertebral destruction has occurred. A suction drain is placed at closure (Fig. 15–1D).

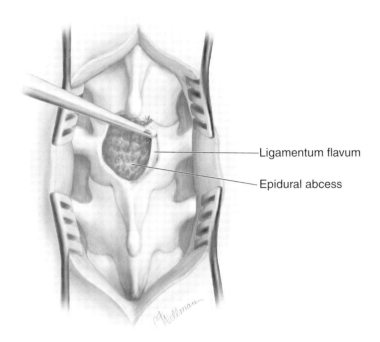

FIGURE 15-1C

The fascia is split in the midline and the muscles are reflected laterally. Laminectomy is performed and ligamentum flavum is elevated until purulence is encountered.

Ligamentum flavum

Epidural abcess

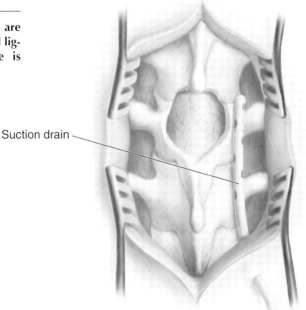

Suction drain

FIGURE 15-1D

Purulent material is debrided and the wound is copiously irrigated. A deep suction drain is placed.

POSTOPERATIVE CARE

Immobilization in a thoracolumbar orthosis may be indicated. Systemic antibiotic therapy is employed for several weeks, depending on cultures obtained during surgery.

OUTCOMES

Improvement in neurologic function should be expected for individuals with incomplete compressive lesions.

COMPLICATIONS

Recurrent infection can occur and may necessitate a secondary operative procedure.

• CORPECTOMY AND INTERBODY FUSION

SUMMARY

Vertebral osteomyelitis is seen infrequently in the thoracic region. Most individuals with this condition are immunocompromised. Tuberculosis has a predilection for this region of the spine. Surgical treatment is indicated for drainage of large abscesses, extensive bony destruction with spinal deformity, extension of the infectious process into the epidural space with neurologic dysfunction, and in patients with persistent symptoms after appropriate antibiotic treatment.

PRESENTATION

Immunocompromised patients are predisposed to this condition. Insidious spinal pain with or without neurologic dysfunction is usual. Fever and constitutional symptoms might be present. Abnormal white blood cell count, sedimentation rate, and C-reactive protein level indicate an infectious process. There may be evidence of a primary infection elsewhere, with seeding to the spine.

NONOPERATIVE CARE

Immobilization and systemic antibiotic therapy may be indicated where bony destruction is not present and neurologic function remains intact. Needle biopsy and culture may be necessary to ascertain the infectious organism and direct antibiotic therapy.

DIAGNOSTIC STUDIES

Plain radiographs permit assessment of spinal alignment and the extent of bony destruction. MRI is the imaging study of choice to show the extent of the infection and the status of neurologic tissues. Radionuclide scanning can be helpful on occasion.

PROCEDURE

CORPECTOMY AND INTERBODY FUSION (FIG. 15–2)

POSITIONING

The procedure is performed through a lateral thoracotomy approach (Fig. 15–2A).

TECHNIQUE

Access is gained through the rib bed superior to the lesion (Fig. 15–2B). Interpleural access is obtained and the site of involvement is identified and confirmed radiographically (Fig. 15–2C). All infected osseous tissue is removed. The epidural

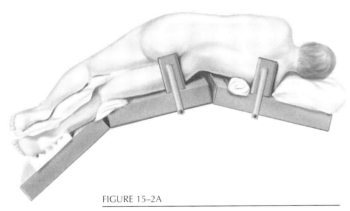

FIGURE 15–2A

INFECTION—CORPECTOMY AND INTERBODY FUSION. The patient is placed in a lateral decubitus position, left side up. Bony prominences are padded.

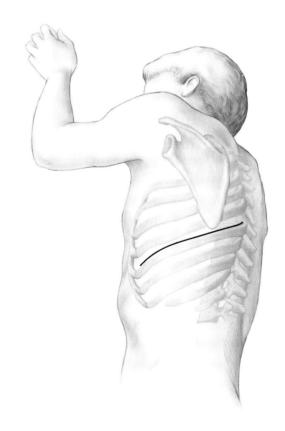

FIGURE 15–2B

A lateral curvilinear incision is made over the appropriate rib.

space is decompressed where indicated. Osseous resection should be carried back to healthy-appearing, bleeding bone. Tricortical iliac crest bone or fibular autograft is placed into the spinal defect (Fig. 15–2D). Instrumentation of a plate-screw configuration may be safely applied if infected tissue has been thoroughly debrided (Fig. 15–2E). Intraoperative cultures are obtained. Antibiotic irrigation is administered during the procedure. A thoracostomy tube is placed before closure.

FIGURE 15-2C

After thoracotomy has been performed, access to the infection is afforded by removal of the head of the rib superior to the lesion. Segmental vessels are ligated as necessary. After radiographic confirmation of the level, infected tissue is removed.

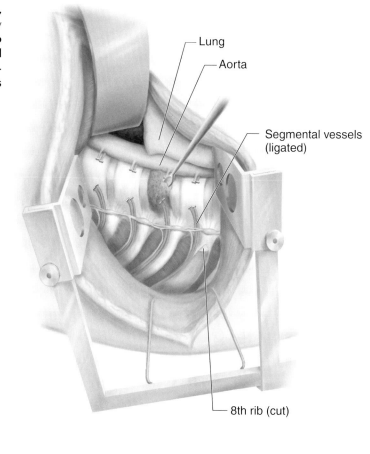

Lung

Aorta

Segmental vessels (ligated)

8th rib (cut)

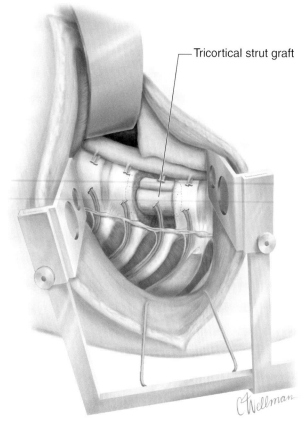

Tricortical strut graft

FIGURE 15-2D

After thorough debridement, a tricortical iliac crest or fibular autograft is placed into the corpectomy defect.

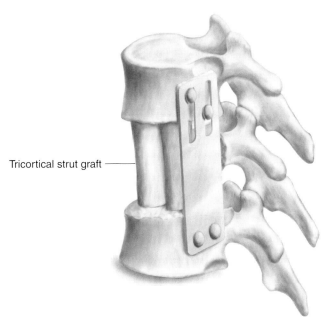

Tricortical strut graft

FIGURE 15-2E

A plate-screw construct can be applied safely during the procedure only after a thorough debridement.

POSTOPERATIVE CARE

A thoracolumbar orthosis is usual. A rehabilitation program is recommended to maximize functional return. Systemic antibiotic therapy is based on culture results.

OUTCOMES

Axial spinal pain should be improved by the procedure and neurologic improvement should be seen in individuals with incomplete deficits.

COMPLICATIONS

Persistent or recurrent infection can occur. Graft dislodgement can be seen and generally requires a repeat operation.

PART III

LOWER CERVICAL SPINE

16

CERVICAL DISK HERNIATION

- ANTERIOR DISK EXCISION AND FUSION
- TWO-LEVEL ANTERIOR DISK EXCISION WITH INSTRUMENTATION
- POSTERIOR DISK EXCISION

- ANTERIOR DISK EXCISION AND FUSION

SUMMARY

Herniation of a disk in the cervical spine is less common than in the lumbar spine. A lateral herniation in the cervical region results in unilateral radicular symptoms. A more centrally located disk might result in myeloradiculopathy. Most herniations occur at C_{5-6} followed by C_{4-5} and C_{6-7}; those are the most mobile levels of the cervical spine. Nonoperative treatment is similar to that for conditions affecting the lumbar spine. Nonsteroidal anti-inflammatory medications, cervical traction, and/or short-term immobilization can be helpful. If symptoms persist, imaging studies might be appropriate. After plain radiographic studies, MRI is the imaging study of choice. The typical posterolateral herniation is best addressed by an anterior approach with total disk excision and interbody fusion using iliac crest bone autograft. Surgical success rates should be in the vicinity of 90% for pain relief and functional improvement.

PRESENTATION

Patients usually present with radicular pain in a dermatomal or sclerotomal distribution. The radicular pattern should correlate with the level of involvement, although there are some variations in anatomic distribution of the nerve roots. Typically, a C_{5-6} disk herniation will compress the C_6 nerve root, resulting in radicular pain in the thumb and forefinger and weakness of the wrist extensors. C_{4-5} disk herniations compress the C_5 nerve root, with resultant weakness of the deltoid and biceps muscles. Pain distribution is more proximal. Disk herniations compressing the C_7 nerve root from the C_{6-7} level result in pain in the ulnar nerve distribution and, on occasion, weakness of the triceps, wrist flexors, and finger flexors. Other levels of disk herniations are rare.

NONOPERATIVE CARE

The natural history of a disk herniation in the cervical region is that of progressive improvement over several weeks, regardless of treatment. Cervical traction can be beneficial. Traction should be applied with the neck flexed forward (i.e., facing the door, if an over-the-door traction unit is to be used). Nonsteroidal anti-inflammatory agents are useful. Physical therapy is of limited benefit. Epidural steroids might provide relief; in many centers, however, there is reluctance to do this procedure due to fear of neurologic injury. The efficacy of oral steroids has not been demonstrated.

DIAGNOSTIC STUDIES

MRI is the study of choice for cervical radicular problems and has supplanted CT or myelogram with CT.

PROCEDURE

ANTERIOR DISK EXCISION AND FUSION (FIG. 16–1)

In patients who do not respond to conservative care, experience intractable pain, or demonstrate progressive neurologic deficit, anterior cervical disk excision with fusion is the procedure of choice for disk herniations occurring in the central and paracentral regions with nerve root compression proximal to the foramen. This is the most common type of cervical disk herniation in the mid- and lower cervical regions.

POSITIONING

The patient is positioned supine. A small roll may be placed in the interscapular region, with the head lying on the operating table or on a horseshoe-type headrest. Halter-type traction removes the mandible from the surgical site (Fig. 16–1A). The procedure is generally performed from the left side, and the bone graft is usually obtained from the anterior iliac crest on the same side. A pad is placed beneath the buttocks to elevate the pelvis for ease in obtaining the bone graft.

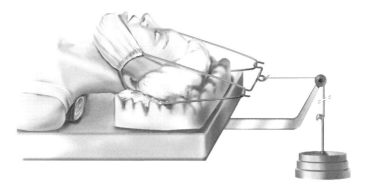

FIGURE 16–1A

ANTERIOR DISK EXCISION AND FUSION. The patient is positioned supine. A roll is placed in the interscapular region to extend the cervical spine. Halter traction is then applied.

TECHNIQUE

The preferred approach is through the left side so as to avoid the recurrent laryngeal nerve with its potentially aberrant course on the right. A transverse incision is made at the appropriate level (generally one fingerbreadth above the clavicle for C_{6-7}, two fingerbreadths above the clavicle for C_{5-6}, and three fingerbreadths above the clavicle for C_{4-5}; Fig. 16–1B). The incision is made in line with the transverse skin lines

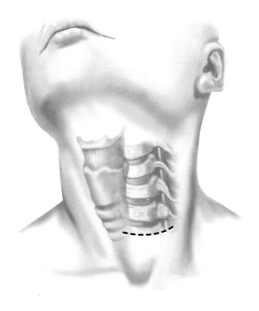

FIGURE 16–1B

A transverse incision is made on the left side at the approximate level of C_6. The location can be confirmed by palpation of Chassaignac's tubercle.

and is 1 to 1.5 inches long. The platysma can be incised transversely or in line with its fibers, thereby exposing the superficial fascia. The fascia is divided and a plane is developed medial to the carotid sheath. The next layer is the deep fascia. The trachea and esophagus are gently retracted to the right side, which exposes the anterior cervical spine. A bent spinal-type needle is placed into the interspace that is thought to be appropriate based on anatomic landmarks and the level of exposure; Chassaignac's tubercle is palpable at C_6. Radiographic confirmation is obtained. Due to anatomic variability, errors at localizing levels are frequent, so no surgery should proceed until the radiograph has been seen. During this period, self-retaining retractors are placed, thereby isolating the area of surgery. A smooth blade is used medially to retract the esophagus and trachea. A pronged retractor can be used beneath the longus coli laterally. After confirmation of the appropriate level, the disk is sharply excised (Fig. 16–1C). Peg retractors may be placed in the adjacent vertebrae and distraction gently applied. Magnification might be desirable in the form of a surgical microscope or headlamp and loupes. Anterior osteophytes, which pre-

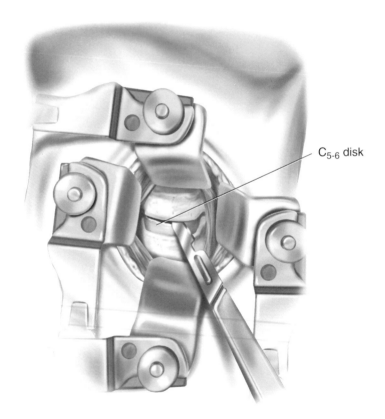

C_{5-6} disk

FIGURE 16-1C

Subcutaneous tissues and platysma are divided, thereby exposing the superficial fascia. The carotid sheath is palpated and taken laterally. The plane deep to the omohyoid muscle is developed bluntly and the trachea and esophagus are retracted medially. Deep fascia is divided. After radiographic localization, the disk is incised.

clude appropriate visualization of the disk space, are removed with Kerrison rongeurs. Residual disk material within the interspace is removed with pituitary forceps (Fig. 16–1D). The posterior longitudinal ligament is visualized. A rent may be apparent in the posterior longitudinal ligament where the disk herniation has occurred. On most occasions, however, a rent is not present and redundant disk tissue is anterior to the posterior longitudinal ligament. Some prefer not to enter the epidural space. If the posterior longitudinal ligament is to be opened, it can be excised with a 1-mm Kerrison rongeur. Resection of osteophytes in the proximal foramen is possible with a small Kerrison rongeur, but care must be taken not to insert too large an instrument or extend too far out into the foramen, where the vertebral artery and nerve roots are located.

After completion of the disk excision, the end-plates of the vertebrae are prepared with a curette or a high-speed burr.

A bone graft, usually 8 to 10 mm in diameter, is obtained from the iliac crest with the use of a dual-bladed saw. Many surgeons will take the bone graft while waiting for the localization radiograph.

The bone graft is contoured appropriately after measuring the depth and width of the interspace. In general, an 8-mm by 12- to 14-mm tricortical iliac crest bone graft is suitable. With distraction applied, the bone graft is inserted, making sure that it does not extend too far posteriorly. Anterior instrumentation may be used (Fig. 16–1E).

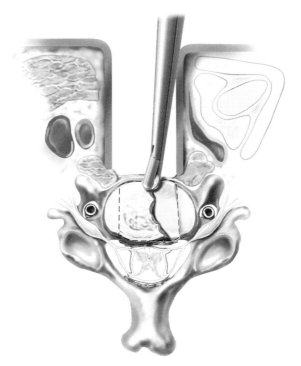

FIGURE 16-1D

A thorough diskectomy is performed. Posterolongitudinal ligament may be opened as desired.

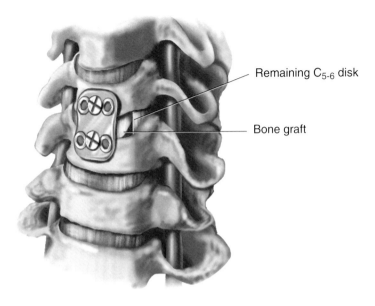

Remaining C$_{5-6}$ disk

Bone graft

FIGURE 16-1E

After disk excision, vertebral end-plates are prepared with a curette or burr. Bone graft is inserted. Anterior instrumentation is then placed.

The peg distractors and other retractors are removed. A radiograph is obtained to ascertain the position of the bone graft and the level of surgery. Anterior instrumentation may be placed, although its usefulness in single-level procedures remains unproven. Closure is routine. A suction drain is placed into the paravertebral space.

POSTOPERATIVE CARE

A soft cervical collar or a more rigid type of cervical collar is used for 6 weeks. Fusion should not be expected until 3 months, but initial consolidation is apparent at 6 weeks.

OUTCOMES

Ninety percent of patients with cervical disk prolapse should be relieved of their radicular symptoms with this procedure. Failures relate to an inappropriate diagnosis, with neck pain exceeding upper extremity pain, or surgery at the wrong level. Rarely, inadequate disk excision and residual nerve root compression occur.

COMPLICATIONS

Dural tears are rare in anterior cervical disk surgery. If they occur, packing with a small amount of collagen sponge usually resolves the problem. Infection is extremely rare–less than 1% with prophylactic antibiotic therapy. Failure of union of the bone graft can occur in up to 15% of cases. The incidence of nonunion is increased in individuals who smoke cigarettes. Vascular complications are rare.

• TWO-LEVEL ANTERIOR DISK EXCISION WITH INSTRUMENTATION

SUMMARY

Rarely, patients present with symptoms that are difficult to ascribe to a single radicular level. Imaging studies might show disk protrusion at two levels. These are usually adjacent. Due to overlapping innervation of nerve roots, the clinician may decide that two levels are involved. In two-level surgery, the incidence of pseudarthrosis is increased and might be exacerbated in individuals who smoke cigarettes or who have poor nutritional status. Evidence suggests that instrumentation with an anterior plate and screws increases the union rate.

PRESENTATION

Symptoms are similar to those of one-level disk herniation with radiculopathy. Upper extremity pain always should exceed neck pain. Neurologic findings are consistent with the level or levels involved.

NONOPERATIVE CARE

As with one-level disease, a trial period of rest, immobilization with a collar, cervical traction, nonsteroidal anti-inflammatory agents, and possibly epidural steroid injections is appropriate. If symptoms persist for more than 6 weeks, surgical treatment may be indicated.

DIAGNOSTIC STUDIES

MRI is the diagnostic study of choice. If this is not available, myelogram with CT can be used.

PROCEDURE

TWO-LEVEL ANTERIOR DISK EXCISION WITH INSTRUMENTATION (FIG. 16–2)

POSITIONING

The supine position is appropriate, with an exposure from the left side. A small pad is placed in the interscapular region. The head can be placed on the operating table or a Mayfield horseshoe-type head holder (Fig. 16–2A). A halter traction device will pull the mandible from the operative field.

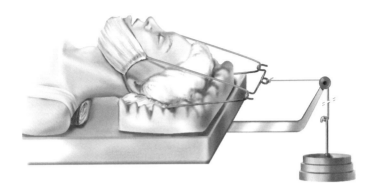

FIGURE 16–2A

TWO-LEVEL ANTERIOR DISK EXCISION WITH INSTRUMEN-TATION. The patient is positioned supine. A roll is placed in the interscapular region to extend the cervical spine. Halter traction is then applied.

TECHNIQUE

The incision is the same as for one-level anterior surgical procedures, with a traditional transverse incision at the appropriate level (Fig. 16–2B). Radiographic confirmation is imperative. After excising most of the disk, the operating microscope can

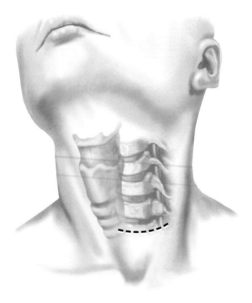

FIGURE 16–2B

A transverse incision is made on the left side at the approximate level of C_6. The location can be confirmed by palpation of Chassaignac's tubercle.

be used to gain access to the posterior longitudinal ligament and epidural space (Fig. 16–2C). The disk herniation is excised back to the posterior longitudinal ligament and, where indicated, the ligament may be resected. Osteophytes in the uncovertebral region also can be removed. Tricortical bone grafts are placed under distraction (Fig. 16–2D). Grafts are generally 8 to 12 mm in height and obtained from the iliac crest, although allograft is employed by some.

Many surgeons feel that fixation with placement of an anterior locking plate is indicated (Fig. 16–2E). Blocks on the drills prevent screw penetration into the spinal canal, with screw length generally being 14 mm. A suction drain is placed into the prevertebral space. Closure is routine, with a plastic-type closure for the skin.

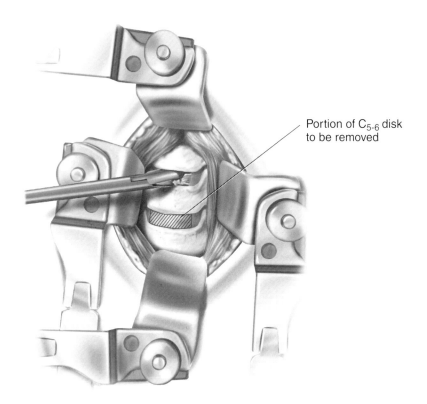

Portion of C$_{5-6}$ disk to be removed

FIGURE 16-2C

Subcutaneous tissues and platysma are divided, thereby exposing the superficial fascia. The carotid sheath is palpated and taken laterally. The plane deep to the omohyoid muscle is developed bluntly and the trachea and esophagus are retracted medially. Deep fascia is divided. After radiographic localization, disks are incised. Thorough diskectomies are performed.

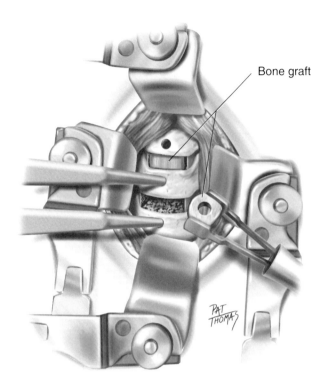

FIGURE 16-2D

For optimal visualization of the disk space, interosseous retractors with distraction can be used. After diskectomy, end-plates are curetted or burred to bleeding bone and bone grafts are placed.

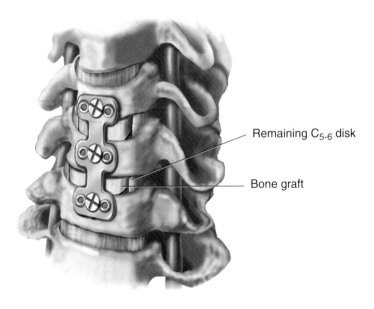

FIGURE 16-2E

Anterior segmental instrumentation is placed.

POSTOPERATIVE CARE

A rigid or soft collar may be used for 6 weeks. Consolidation of the fusion is expected at 3 to 6 months. Return to full function is expected at 3 months.

OUTCOMES

Functional improvement is expected in 85% of patients. Success rates are somewhat lower than with one-level disease due to the difficulties in diagnosis and the more extensive nature of the surgery.

COMPLICATIONS

Dural tears are rare. Infections occur in less than 1%. Nonunion can occur in up to 30% of cases but is decreased by the use of internal fixation. Spinal cord injury due to technical factors is extremely rare.

• POSTERIOR DISK EXCISION

SUMMARY

Posterior disk excision may be used for lateral disk herniations in the cervical spine. Such herniations result in unilateral radiculopathy. Imaging studies will show intraforaminal compression. Although not a common procedure in the past, this has become more prominent due to current concepts of limited access surgery and use of the operating microscope. The posterior approach is most useful for a disk herniation in the axilla of the nerve root. Care must be taken during the surgical treatment to avoid compression of the spinal cord or excessive traction on the nerve root.

PRESENTATION

Unilateral radiculopathy is the presenting symptom. Neck pain is usually minimal. Failure of nonoperative treatment may be an indication for surgery in the presence of incapacitating symptoms. Neurologic findings correlate with the level of nerve root compression.

NONOPERATIVE CARE

Nonoperative care involves brief periods of rest, immobilization with a cervical collar, nonsteroidal anti-inflammatory agents, cervical traction, and, on occasion, epidural steroids or selective nerve root block.

DIAGNOSTIC STUDIES

MRI remains the imaging modality of choice for all cervical disk problems. Where not available, myelogram CT can be used as a substitute.

PROCEDURE

POSTERIOR DISK EXCISION (FIG. 16–3)

POSITIONING

The patient is placed in a prone position or semi-sitting with skull fixation (Fig. 16–3A). In the prone position, halter traction may be substituted.

TECHNIQUE

It is best to obtain a localization radiograph with a marker before the skin incision. A small, 0.5- to 1-inch long skin incision is made in the paravertebral area approximately one fingerbreadth parallel to the midline (Fig. 16–3B). The incision is carried down to the area of the facet joint (Fig. 16–3C). A high-speed burr is used to resect bone. A circular, 1-cm window is created (Fig. 16–3D). Use of a diamond-type burr will minimize the risk of a dural tear on entry into the epidural space. The nerve root is identified, as is a small vascular complex within the axilla. The disk herniation

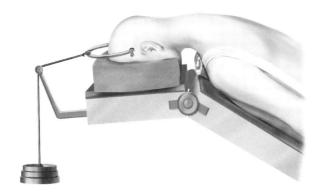

FIGURE 16–3A

POSTERIOR DISK EXCISION. The patient is positioned prone, with the neck slightly flexed. Bony prominences, including orbits, are well padded. Skeletal traction is employed.

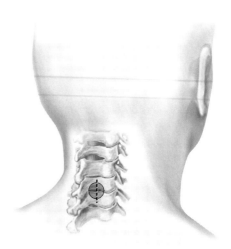

FIGURE 16–3B

A small skin incision is made one fingerbreadth lateral to the midline over the desired level.

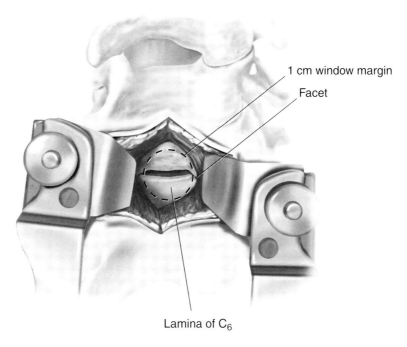

1 cm window margin

Facet

Lamina of C$_6$

FIGURE 16-3C

Muscles are divided bluntly and retracted to expose the inter-laminar space. Self-retaining retractors are inserted.

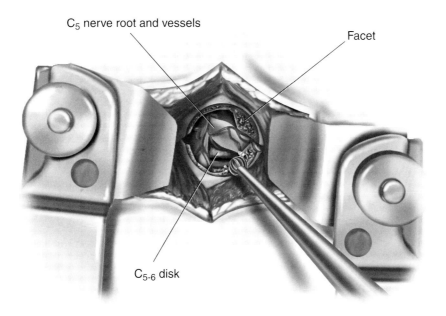

C$_5$ nerve root and vessels

Facet

C$_{5-6}$ disk

FIGURE 16-3D

A high-speed burr is used to create a circular 1-cm window. The nerve root crossing the field obliquely is identified.

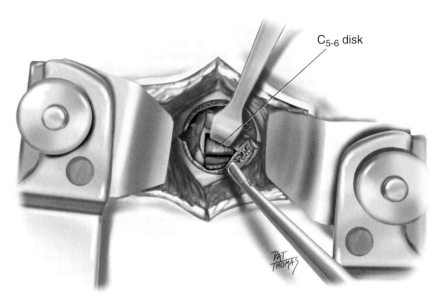

FIGURE 16-3E
_____

The vascular leash overlying the disk is coagulated with bipolar electrocautery. The disk herniation is gently dissected free and removed.

should be apparent just inferior to the exiting nerve root lateral to the spinal cord (Fig. 16–3E). The vessel leash should be coagulated with bipolar electrocautery. The disk herniation is gently teased free with a neural dissector and removed with a micropituitary forceps. The area should be explored for any other fragments of disk material. A limited foraminotomy can be performed with Kerrison rongeurs. A drain is optional. Closure is routine.

POSTOPERATIVE CARE

Limited immobilization and a soft cervical collar are generally employed for a period of one to two weeks. After this, restricted activity is maintained up to six weeks.

OUTCOMES

For properly selected patients, the surgical success rate should be approximately 90%. Failures relate to diagnostic error, with inaccessibility of a more centrally located disk tissue. Outcomes are similar with microscopic procedures and so-called percutaneous speculum-type procedures.

COMPLICATIONS

Nerve root damage can occur from excessive traction on the nerve root. Similar problems can occur with the spinal cord but are rare. The problem of postoperative bleeding can be obviated by use of bipolar cautery in the nerve root axilla.

17

STENOSIS

- ANTERIOR DECOMPRESSION AND FUSION
- POSTERIOR LAMINECTOMY
- POSTERIOR LAMINAPLASTY

- ANTERIOR DECOMPRESSION AND FUSION

SUMMARY

Cervical spinal stenosis usually results in myelopathy and radiculopathy. In a straight or kyphotic spine with "draping" of the cord, an anterior procedure is indicated. Vertebral corpectomy with excision of bone to the lateral aspect of the spinal canal is appropriate. Traditionally, anterior excision has been limited to three vertebral bodies with posterior surgery customary for four or more segments; this is controversial. A structural bone graft is necessary to replace the vertebral segments removed for anterior spinal canal decompression. For two or three segments, a tricortical iliac crest bone graft is appropriate. Autograft or allograft fibula can be used for more extensive vertebral body resections.

PRESENTATION

Cervical myelopathy is a result of spinal cord compression. It generally manifests itself in global sensory and motor disturbances. Upper motor neuron findings are common, with distal hyperreflexia, clonus, and Babinski and Hoffman signs, depending on the severity of spinal cord compression.

NONOPERATIVE CARE

The natural history of cervical myelopathy is that of improvement in approximately one-third of patients, no change in one-third of patients, and progression in the remaining one-third. The risk of neurologic deterioration and paralysis is small. As such, emergent surgical procedures are rare.

Nonsteroidal anti-inflammatory medication may be slightly beneficial. Oral steroids have not been proven to be effective. Epidural steroid injection is controversial but might be helpful in some individuals. Traction is usually of minimal benefit. Physical therapy is generally not helpful.

DIAGNOSTIC STUDIES

MRI is the procedure of choice, with myelogram and CT as an alternative. Both will permit diagnosis of anterior spinal cord compression and might show evidence of parenchymal changes within the spinal cord or syringomyelia.

PROCEDURE

ANTERIOR DECOMPRESSION AND FUSION (FIG. 17–1)

POSITIONING

The procedure is performed in a supine position. Halter traction or skull-tong traction can be used (Fig. 17–1A).

TECHNIQUE

For one- or two-segment disease, a transverse incision is appropriate; for more extensive procedures, an oblique incision along the anterior border of the ster-

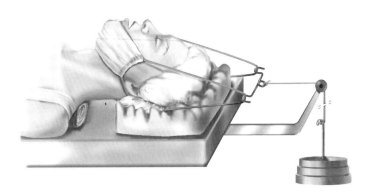

FIGURE 17–1A

STENOSIS-ANTERIOR DECOMPRESSION AND FUSION. The patient is placed supine, with a head halter or skeletal traction in place.

nocleidomastoid is used (Fig. 17–1B). Dissection is carried medial to the carotid sheath down to the anterior aspect of the spinal column. A confirmatory radiograph is obtained with a needle placed into the intervertebral disk space. Self-retaining retractors are placed. With a rongeur, excessive osteophytes are removed. A high-speed burr is then used to excise bone and develop a trough through the extent of the area to be decompressed (Fig. 17–1C). Residual posterior

FIGURE 17–1B

A transverse or oblique incision can be used. In this case, for two-level disease, a standard transverse approach is shown.

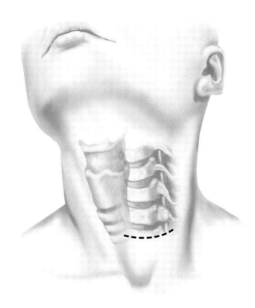

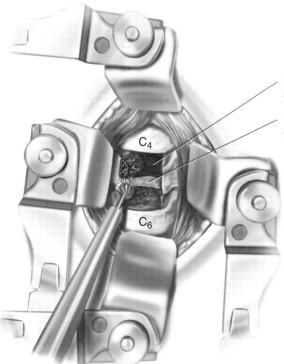

Remnant of cortical shell of C$_5$

Posterior remnant of C$_{5-6}$ disk

C$_4$

C$_6$

FIGURE 17-1C

Dissection is carried medial to the sternocleidomastoid, with division of several fibers of omohyoid. The carotid is taken laterally and the trachea and esophagus medially. The potential space anterior to the cervical spine is entered. After radiographic confirmation of the appropriate level, corpectomy and diskectomy are performed.

bone can be removed with a small Kerrison rongeur and straight and angled curettes (Fig. 17–1D). Attempts should not be made to remove small plaques adherent to the dura. Limited foraminotomies can be performed. Bone grafting is always necessary with distraction used before placement of the bone graft (Fig. 17–1E). This achieves a semblance of restoration of lordosis. Some surgeons place a bridging plate fixation device anteriorly, others use a small buttress-type plate at the superior and inferior aspects of the graft to hold it in place, and others opt for no fixation. Closure over a suction drain is routine. When structural integrity is questionable, a halo device may be used postoperatively. Otherwise, rigid collar immobilization is indicated.

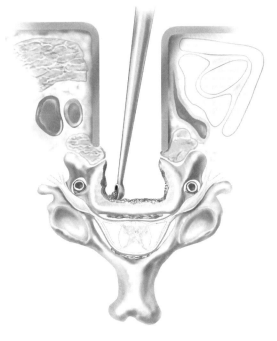

FIGURE 17-1D

Decompression is carried posterior to the posterior longitudinal ligament. Limited foraminotomies may be performed. The posterior longitudinal ligament need not be opened.

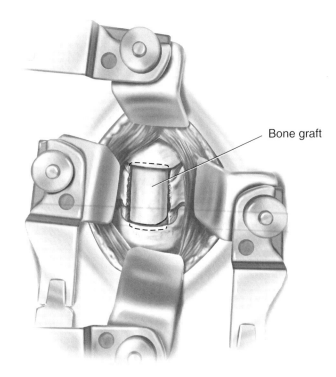

Bone graft

FIGURE 17-1E

After corpectomy, troughs are created rostrally and caudally and a bone graft is placed.

POSTOPERATIVE CARE

Postoperative care depends on adequacy of structural fixation at the time of surgery. Choices for immobilization range from a hard cervical collar to a halo device. Rehabilitation might be indicated for patients with severe myelopathic symptoms so as to maximize postoperative fixation.

OUTCOMES

With appropriate indications and adequate surgical technique, some improvement is expected immediately. That improvement is followed by progressive improvement over the short and intermediate terms. Approximately 75% to 85% of patients will have some relief, most notably in upper extremity pain and function. There are better results in those with less preoperative symptomatology.

COMPLICATIONS

Graft dislodgment can occur and generally is related to inadequate structural fixation at the time of surgery. If this occurs, repeat surgery and consideration of supplemental fixation in the form of a plate and screws or external halo fixation may be appropriate. Dural tears are rare. If they occur, they can be managed expectantly. Infection occurs rarely. Graft nonunion can occur in 15% to 30% of cases.

• POSTERIOR LAMINECTOMY

SUMMARY

Cervical spondylosis or congenital spinal stenosis with superimposed spondylosis can cause myelopathy or myeloradiculopathy. Most often, this occurs in elderly patients with some ankylosis of the spine. Those patients may have preservation of the cervical lordosis. Posterior laminectomy is a surgical option for such individuals. Alternative procedures to treat myelopathy are anterior decompression and fusion for patients with straight or kyphotic spines or posterior laminaplasty for younger individuals in whom lordosis is preserved.

PRESENTATION

Patients present with cervical myelopathies: distal upper motor neuron signs and, on occasion, elements of radiculopathy due to foraminal or preforaminal stenosis. Motor and sensory disturbances predominate.

NONOPERATIVE CARE

As with other forms of cervical myelopathy, understanding the natural history is important. Some benefit has been reported from rest, immobilization with a cervical collar, cervical traction, and epidural steroid injection. Oral steroids are generally of minimal or no benefit. Surgical treatment is considered for progressive neurologic deterioration or significant functional impairment.

DIAGNOSTIC STUDIES

MRI is the diagnostic imaging study of choice. Myelogram with CT may be substituted in patients who are claustrophobic or in whom MRI is contraindicated.

PROCEDURE

POSTERIOR LAMINECTOMY (FIG. 17–2)

POSITIONING

The procedure is performed through a posterior approach (Fig. 17–2A). A prone position or a modified sitting position is used. Skull-tong or halter traction is used to position the head appropriately.

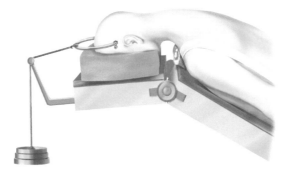

FIGURE 17–2A

STENOSIS-POSTERIOR LAMINECTOMY. The patient is positioned prone, with skeletal or halter traction. The neck is flexed slightly to diminish lordosis and improve access to the spine.

TECHNIQUE

A longitudinal incision is made in the midline (Fig. 17–2B). Muscular elements are dissected free of the posterior aspect of the spine and self-retaining retractors are placed. As is the case in procedures on the lumbar spine, extensive decompression is preferred so as not to miss elements of stenosis (Fig. 17–2C). Most commonly, the disease extends from C_{3-4} through C_{6-7}. The spinous processes are excised (Fig. 17–2D). The epidural space is entered gently and the posterior elements are excised with the use of power instruments or Kerrison rongeurs. Bipolar cautery is used to control epidural venous bleeding. Limited foraminotomy may be performed. Care should be taken not to apply excessive pressure or suction to the dura itself. Closure is routine over a small, deep drain to avoid a postoperative epidural hematoma.

FIGURE 17–2B

A longitudinal incision is made over the areas to be decompressed.

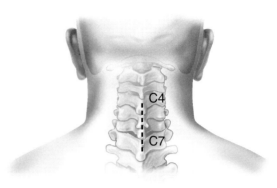

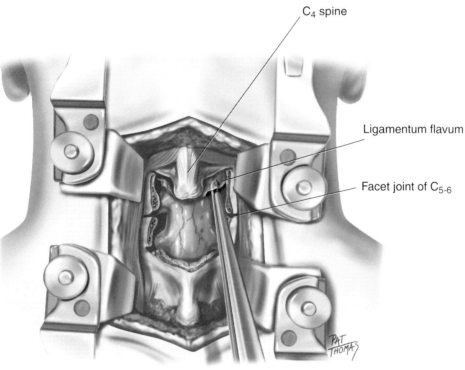

C₄ spine

Ligamentum flavum

Facet joint of C₅₋₆

FIGURE 17-2C

A standard posterior exposure is performed. Muscles are retracted laterally to the facets. Laminectomies and foraminotomies are performed.

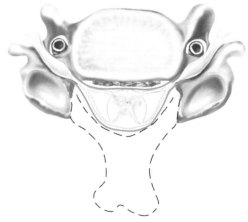

FIGURE 17-2D

The extent of decompression is shown.

POSTOPERATIVE CARE

Postoperative immobilization with a soft cervical collar for 6 weeks is appropriate. Patients should be ambulatory soon after surgery.

OUTCOMES

With appropriately selected patients, 75% to 85% improvement is expected.

COMPLICATIONS

The most feared complication of cervical laminectomy is that of postoperative kyphosis. Muscular attachments at C_2 must be preserved to avoid it. Kyphosis should not occur in elderly patients with extensive spondylosis and ankylosis at multiple levels. In younger individuals, particularly those who are not skeletally mature, this is a serious risk. Individuals with subluxation should be instrumented at the time of the procedure. Dural tears are rare but should be dealt with intraoperatively. Residual myelopathy might be the result of persistent anterior spinal cord compression, which may necessitate a secondary anterior procedure.

• POSTERIOR LAMINAPLASTY

SUMMARY

Laminaplasty is appropriate for individuals with lordotic cervical spines with symptoms of congenital stenosis and/or ossification of the posterior longitudinal ligament (OPLL). The Japanese, in whom OPLL is relatively common, have popularized this procedure. It is rarely indicated in individuals without OPLL or congenital stenosis. Theoretical advantages of the procedure are the prevention of postoperative kyphosis and preservation of motion. The latter advantage has not been realized.

PRESENTATION

Patients present with myelopathy. Upper and lower motor neuron symptoms might be present. A candidate for laminaplasty must have preservation of the cervical lordosis.

NONOPERATIVE CARE

Nonoperative care is similar to that described for cervical myelopathy. This includes observation, immobilization in a cervical orthosis, nonsteroidal anti-inflammatory agents, and, on occasion, epidural steroid injection.

DIAGNOSTIC STUDIES

As with all other cervical conditions, MRI is the diagnostic imaging study of choice. Myelogram with CT is an alternative for those who cannot tolerate MRI or those in whom it is contraindicated.

PROCEDURE

POSTERIOR LAMINAPLASTY (FIG. 17–3)

POSITIONING

The patient is positioned prone, with the head elevated. A semi-sitting position also can be used (Fig. 17–3A).

TECHNIQUE

A midline posterior incision is made (Fig. 17–3B). Self-retaining retractors are placed after incision and retraction of the muscles. With the use of a high-speed burr, troughs are placed at the lateral aspects of the laminae in the segments to be win-

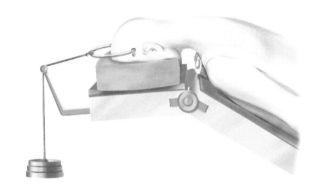

FIGURE 17–3A

STENOSIS-POSTERIOR LAMINOPLASTY. The patient is positioned prone, with skull-tong traction. The neck is flexed to reduce lordosis and improve access to the spine.

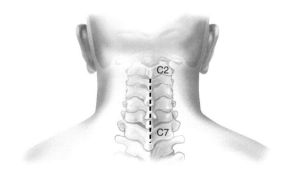

FIGURE 17–3B

A standard posterior midline incision is made.

dowed (Fig. 17–3C). This generally is undertaken from just below C$_2$ to the C$_{6-7}$ level. The trough is extended into the epidural space with a small Kerrison rongeur on the side to be reflected. This is usually the side with symptoms of radiculopathy. The contralateral side is thinned so that, with gradual elevation of the spinous processes, the "door" can be opened. Elevation of 1 cm on the "open-door" side is desirable. Tips of the spinous processes may be resected to prevent the muscles from compressing the elevated posterior elements. Drill holes are placed in the spinous processes of the elevated segments and nonresorbable sutures are extended into the facet joint capsules of the hinge side and tied tightly (Fig. 17–3D). Some difficulties have been experienced keeping the laminaplasty "door" open, and a variety of techniques have been described to prevent that. One such technique uses a bone graft to lodge the "door" open (Fig. 17–3E). Small bits of bone obtained from the spinous processes can be placed into the trough of the hinged side to fibrose or ankylose it. During the procedure, bleeding after elevation of the door is frequently encountered. Bleeding can be controlled with bipolar cautery, gentle packing, or coagulation devices. A drain is usually employed. Closure is routine.

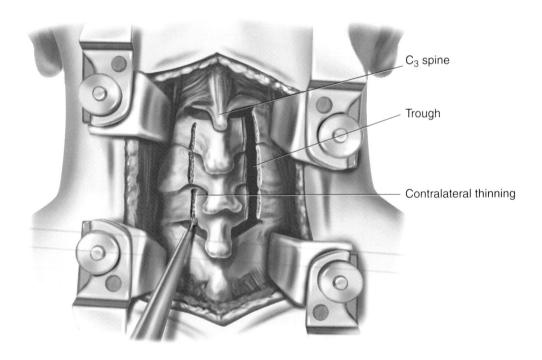

C$_3$ spine

Trough

Contralateral thinning

FIGURE 17-3C

Dissection is carried laterally to the facets. A trough is created unilaterally with a high-speed burr. On the contralateral side, a full-thickness trough is created with a Kerrison rongeur. The "door" is then opened toward the side of the initial trough.

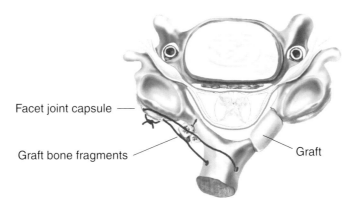

Facet joint capsule

Graft bone fragments

Graft

FIGURE 17-3D

After the door has been opened, a bone graft is placed to maintain canal expansion.

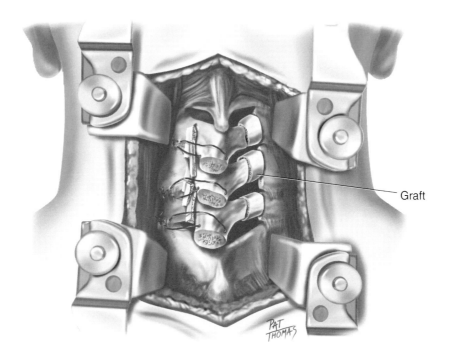

Graft

FIGURE 17-3E

Drill holes are placed in the spinous processes of the elevated segments and nonabsorbable sutures or wires are placed between the spinous process and the hinge-side facet capsules. Local autograft also can be placed in the trough of the hinge side.

POSTOPERATIVE CARE

A cervical orthosis can be employed for 6 weeks. Limited motion of the neck is permitted for 3 months.

OUTCOMES

Results generally are similar to those with laminectomy, although stiffness of the neck is frequent due to the extensive nature of the procedure.

COMPLICATIONS

Excessive bleeding frequently occurs when the "door" is elevated. Stiffness of the neck is common postoperatively. With the routine procedure not employing "props" to keep the door open, closure can occur, necessitating re-exploration and, on occasion, conversion of the procedure to a laminectomy.

18

INSTABILITY AND STENOSIS

- ## POSTERIOR DECOMPRESSION WITH WIRED BONE GRAFT
- ## POSTERIOR DECOMPRESSION WITH LATERAL MASS PLATE FUSION

- ## POSTERIOR DECOMPRESSION WITH WIRED BONE GRAFT

SUMMARY

Some patients will present with instability of the cervical spine associated with cervical spinal stenosis. The stenosis is manifested as a myelopathic syndrome with or without radicular pain. The pathology is related to degenerative change with subluxation at one or more levels or an inflammatory condition such as rheumatoid arthritis, with resultant soft tissue abnormalities and vertebral subluxation. The effect is that of absolute stenosis (osteophytic or ligamentous encroachment into the spinal canal) or relative stenosis (spinal cord impingement due to subluxation). Patients present with neck pain, spinal cord, or nerve root symptoms. Lordosis usually is maintained in this condition. The surgical procedure of choice is decompressive laminectomy in conjunction with lateral mass arthrodesis.

PRESENTATION

Neck pain due to instability is common in conjunction with neurologic symptoms due to spinal cord and nerve root compression. Upper motor neuron and lower motor neuron symptoms might be present, with the latter relating to radicular syndromes.

NONOPERATIVE CARE

Patients with mild to moderate symptoms can be managed with immobilization in a cervical orthosis. Rigid orthotic devices are poorly tolerated. A soft collar will suffice. Nonsteroidal anti-inflammatory agents and diminished activity can help. Epidural steroid injection might be of some benefit in selected patients.

DIAGNOSTIC STUDIES

Plain radiographs permit assessment of cervical lordosis and the degree of subluxation in a neutral position. Flexion–extension radiographs are very important to establish what elements of dynamic instability exist. MRI is useful to analyze the neural elements and assess any changes in the spinal cord. Myelography with CT is an adjunctive study that can add information with regard to nerve root compression, particularly in the foraminal regions.

PROCEDURE

POSTERIOR DECOMPRESSION WITH WIRED BONE GRAFT (FIG. 18–1)

POSITIONING

This is a posterior procedure performed in the prone position. The head is placed on a horseshoe head holder. Traction may be applied with skull tongs, if desired (Fig. 18–1A).

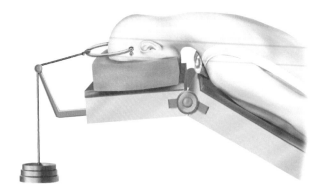

FIGURE 18–1A

INSTABILITY AND STENOSIS-POSTERIOR DECOMPRESSION WITH WIRED BONE GRAFT. The patient is positioned prone, with skull-tong traction. The neck is flexed to reduce lordosis and improve access to the spine.

TECHNIQUE

The incision is midline (Fig. 18–1B). Self-retaining retractors are used. A confirming radiograph is used to localize the levels of the surgery. The spinous processes at the levels involved are removed (Fig. 18–1C). The epidural space is entered. Laminectomy is performed with Kerrison rongeurs. Dissection is carried out to the laminar–facet junction. Epidural venous bleeding is controlled with bipolar cautery, packing, and coagulating agents. Drill holes are placed into the facets. This is best

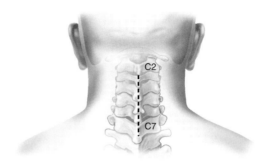

FIGURE 18–1B

A standard posterior midline incision is made.

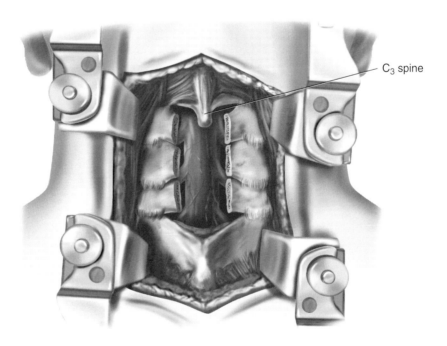

FIGURE 18-1C

Muscles are reflected laterally to the facets. A laminectomy is performed.

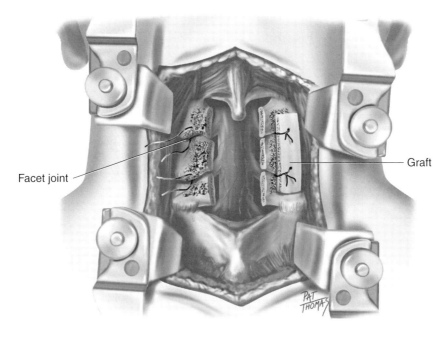

FIGURE 18-1D

After laminectomy, drill holes are made in the facets. A wire or cable is passed through and corticocancellous bone graft is wired in segmentally.

accomplished by placing a small elevator into the facet joint itself and using power instruments to drill in the middle portion of the facet. A wire or cable is passed. This procedure is performed at all levels to be fused.

Strips of corticocancellous bone graft are obtained from the iliac crest and placed over the decorticated posterior elements (Fig. 18–1D). Supplementary morsels of cancellous bone graft may be placed into the facets. Wires are passed through the facets and through drill holes in the graft and gently tightened down, securing the onlay bone graft. A drain is placed and closure is routine.

POSTOPERATIVE CARE

Immobilization in a rigid cervical orthosis is appropriate. Halo immobilization generally is not necessary. Immobilization is used for 3 months to ensure graft consolidation and arthrodesis.

OUTCOMES

The outcome with regard to neurologic improvement should be similar to those with a laminectomy. Stiffness of the neck as a result of the procedure is unavoidable.

COMPLICATIONS

Dural tears are rare. Epidural venous bleeding can occur but should be controlled with bipolar cautery, packing, and coagulating agents. Most patients note restricted cervical spine motion.

• POSTERIOR DECOMPRESSION WITH LATERAL MASS PLATE FUSION

SUMMARY

This procedure is indicated for cervical spinal stenosis with instability. Neurologic symptoms of myelopathy and radiculopathy are the most usual presentation. Subluxation on radiographs is an indication for arthrodesis. Plate fixation is an alternative to wired bone graft.

PRESENTATION

Myelopathy results in upper motor neuron symptoms, with weakness and sensory disturbances in the upper and lower extremities, depending on the level of involvement. Radiculopathy might be present due to foraminal encroachment from vertebral subluxation.

NONOPERATIVE CARE

Orthotic immobilization of the neck is appropriate. Nonsteroidal anti-inflammatory agents, rest, and, on occasion, epidural steroid injection might be beneficial. With persistent symptoms, surgical intervention is indicated.

DIAGNOSTIC STUDIES

Plain radiographs show the alignment of the spine and the relative position of the vertebrae in the neutral position. Lateral flexion–extension radiographs will indicate any evidence of a dynamic instability. MRI shows evidence of neural compression and the status of the spinal cord and other neural elements. Myelogram with CT is an adjunctive procedure that might be beneficial for assessment of foraminal compression of the nerve roots.

PROCEDURE

POSTERIOR DECOMPRESSION WITH LATERAL MASS PLATE FUSION (FIG. 18-2)

POSITIONING

The procedure is performed with the patient in the prone position (Fig. 18–2A). The head is placed on a horseshoe headrest. Skull-tong traction is optional.

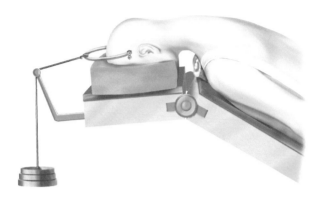

FIGURE 18-2A

POSTERIOR DECOMPRESSION WITH LATERAL MASS PLATE FUSION. The patient is positioned prone, with skull-tong traction. The neck is flexed to reduce lordosis and improve access to the spine.

TECHNIQUE

The procedure is performed through a midline posterior approach (Fig. 18–2B). After exposure of the elements and placement of self-retaining retractors, a confirming radiograph is obtained to localize the level of surgery. Spinous processes are excised and the epidural space is identified through the inferior interlaminar region (Fig. 18–2C). Laminectomy is performed with Kerrison rongeurs, occasionally with the assistance of a high-speed burr. Laminectomy is carried to the lateral extent of the spinal canal. Limited foraminotomies may be performed. Bleeding is controlled with bipolar cautery, packing, and coagulating agents.

The lateral masses and facet joints are gently decorticated with a high-speed burr. Bone graft is placed. Drill holes are placed in the mid-portion of the inferior facets, angling approximately 30 degrees upward and 15 degrees lateral. In this way, contact with neural and vascular structures is avoided. An appropriately sized plate is placed and affixed (Fig. 18–2D). Screws are generally 14 to 16 mm long. A drain is placed before closure.

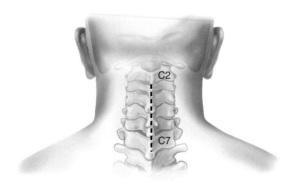

FIGURE 18-2B

A standard posterior midline incision is made.

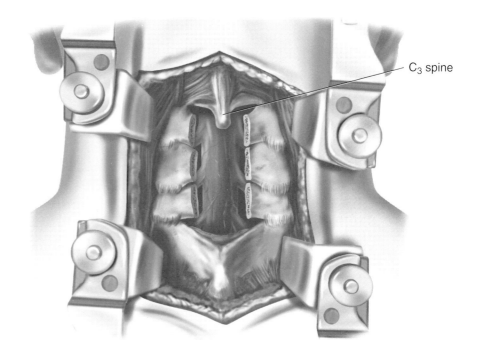

FIGURE 18-2C

Muscles are reflected laterally to the facets. A laminectomy is performed.

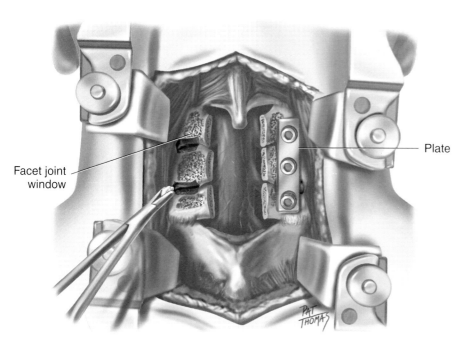

FIGURE 18-2D

Lateral masses and facets are decorticated with a burr and bone graft is placed. Holes are drilled in the mid-portion of the inferior facets at an angle of 30 degrees rostrally and 15 degrees laterally. An appropriately–sized plate is fixed to the spine with the requisite number of screws.

POSTOPERATIVE CARE

Immobilization with a cervical orthosis is appropriate and should be maintained for 3 months. Progressive ambulation and activity are instituted.

OUTCOMES

Improvement is anticipated in 75% to 85% of individuals. Stiffness of the neck is anticipated.

COMPLICATIONS

Dural tears occasionally can occur and be controlled by direct repair and/or packing. Intraoperative bleeding is controlled with electrocautery and packing. Pseudarthrosis is uncommon.

19

FRACTURES

- FACET DISLOCATION: POSTERIOR STABILIZATION
- C$_5$ BURST FRACTURE: ANTERIOR DECOMPRESSION AND FUSION

- FACET DISLOCATION: POSTERIOR STABILIZATION

SUMMARY

Instability of the cervical spine usually occurs as a result of trauma, with disruption of the ligamentous and capsular structures of the facet joints. Disruption is manifested in a unilateral facet subluxation, unilateral facet fracture–dislocation, or a bilateral facet dislocation. Neurologic sequelae relate to the severity of the injury and range from no neurologic deficit to unilateral radiculopathy to spinal cord injury. Because the injury is posterior in nature, surgery is best performed from the posterior approach. Nonoperative measures are generally not successful unless the injury is predominantly osseous.

PRESENTATION

Trauma is usually the precipitating event. Neurologic injury in the form of nerve root compression or spinal cord injury might be present.

NONOPERATIVE CARE

Nonoperative measures are generally not successful, and surgical treatment is indicated when angular instability exceeds 11 degrees or translational instability exceeds 3.5 mm. If those criteria are not met, consideration can be given to immobilization in a cervical orthosis for 2 to 3 weeks followed by repeat flexion–extension radiographs to assess spinal stability.

DIAGNOSTIC STUDIES

Bony abnormalities and the resting alignment of the cervical spine are shown on plain radiographs. Supplementary flexion–extension lateral radiographs will show any occult instability. If necessary, CT helps to define bony anatomy. MRI is the study of choice for imaging neural elements and ruling out unrecognized disk herniation. Often, all of these studies are indicated.

PROCEDURE

FACET DISLOCATION: POSTERIOR STABILIZATION (FIG. 19–1)

POSITIONING

Since this is a posterior injury, the procedure is performed through a posterior approach. Skull-tong traction or halo immobilization is generally utilized (Fig. 19–1A).

TECHNIQUE

A midline approach is used (Fig. 19–1B). Dissection should be limited to the area of injury to avoid creating iatrogenic injury at other levels. The subluxated area is easily identified. If the injury is acute, general reduction is indicated. Neural dissectors or elevators and a towel clip are used to reduce the facet joints (Fig. 19–1C). A wire or cable is inserted through the posterior aspects of the spinous processes and gently tightened to hold the reduction in place. An oblique wire extending from the spinous process below to the inferior facet at the injury site

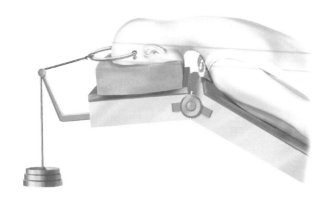

FIGURE 19–1A

FRACTURE-FACET DISLOCATION AND POSTERIOR STABILIZATION. The patient is positioned prone, with the spine at an attitude of minimal to moderate flexion. Skull traction is carefully applied.

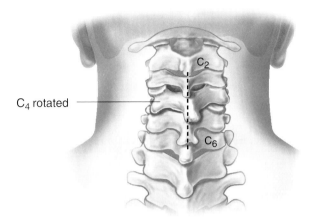

FIGURE 19–1B

A standard midline approach is centered over the level of the fracture.

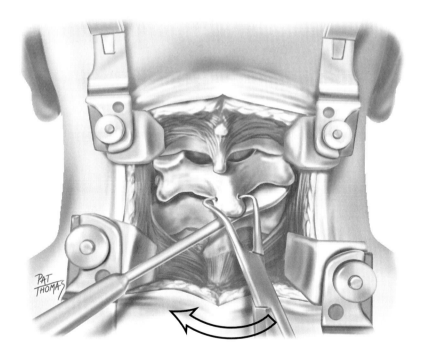

FIGURE 19-1C

Posterior musculature is carefully dissected. The supraspinous and intraspinous ligaments rostral and caudal to the level of the injury should not be disrupted. When the injury has been identified, reduction is performed.

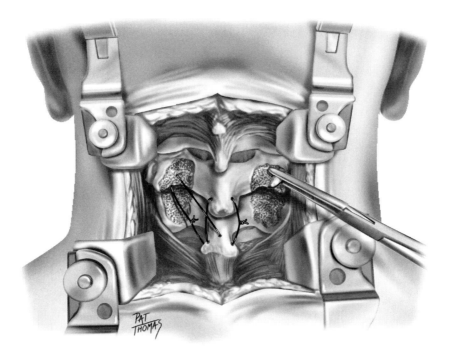

FIGURE 19-1D

After reduction, spinous process wiring is performed, usually with an oblique wire to prevent resubluxation.

may supplement the fixation (Fig. 19–1D). Lateral mass plating is another fixation option. Decortication with a burr is performed over the exposed facet joints, and posterior elements and bone graft are laid in place. An interpositional bone graft between the spinous processes may be used. Morcellized bone graft from the posterior iliac crest is applied to the decorticated posterior elements. Drainage is optional. Closure is routine.

POSTOPERATIVE CARE

Immobilization in a cervical orthosis is recommended for 6 to 12 weeks. A halo device is not necessary unless there is also injury to the anterior elements.

OUTCOMES

Stabilization is achieved and maintained in most cases. Neurologic recovery is related to the severity of the initial deficit.

COMPLICATIONS

The usual complications of a dural injury, spinal cord injury and failure of union, occur in this condition but are rare.

• C₅ BURST FRACTURE: ANTERIOR DECOMPRESSION AND FUSION

SUMMARY

Burst injuries of the anterior column of the cervical spine are relatively common and often catastrophic, with frequent neurologic injury. They most commonly occur in the mid-cervical region, with C_5 predominating, followed by C_4. With disruption of the posterior aspect of the vertebral body, intrusion of bone into the spinal canal and injury of the spinal cord can occur. Intrusion might be incomplete or complete. Surgical treatment is frequently performed to address instability and neural compromise.

PRESENTATION

These are acute injuries of an axial-loading nature commonly due to motor vehicle accidents and sporting injuries. The neurologic deficit corresponds to the degree of spinal canal compromise sustained at the time of injury. Incomplete lesions result in partial paralysis and sensory disturbance distal to the lesion. Complete lesions result in immediate absence of neurologic function distal to the level of injury. Incomplete lesions are prone to improvement regardless of the form of treatment. Complete lesions generally do not improve, although some "root escape" can occur over time.

The neurologic situation is apparent, with the neurologic level of injury named for the last functioning neurologic segment for complete injuries. A variety of incomplete neurologic lesions have been described, such as anterior, central, and posterior cord syndromes and the Brown–Séquard syndrome. A detailed examination is necessary at the time of presentation to predict prognosis and help in treatment selection.

NONOPERATIVE CARE

On rare occasions, when other injuries or medical conditions preclude surgical intervention, some burst injuries can be treated with traction immobilization. Surgery is indicated most often in incomplete lesions. Complete lesions usually are not improved by decompressive procedures. An optional treatment for the instability, however, might be surgical stabilization.

DIAGNOSTIC STUDIES

Plain radiographs assess overall anatomic alignment of the spine and the features of the injury. CT is indicated to diagnose osseous injury, and MRI is valuable to assess the condition of the neural elements. Often, all of these studies are necessary.

PROCEDURE

C$_5$ BURST FRACTURE: ANTERIOR DECOMPRESSION AND FUSION (FIG. 19–2)

POSITIONING

This is an anterior procedure and, on occasion, an anterior and posterior procedure if gross instability exists. The anterior procedure is performed through the traditional supine approach. Skull-tong traction or a halo device is usually in place at the beginning of the procedure (Fig. 19–2A).

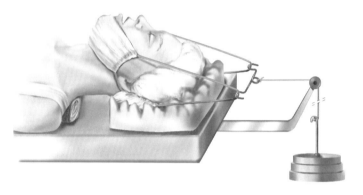

FIGURE 19–2A

C$_5$ BURST FRACTURE-ANTERIOR DECOMPRESSION AND FUSION. The patient is placed supine, with skull-tong or head-halter traction.

TECHNIQUE

For one-level disease, a transverse-type incision can be used (Fig. 19–2B). Such an incision is best approached from the left side. For more extensive surgery, an oblique-type incision along the anterior aspect of the sternocleidomastoid is recommended. Dissection is carried medial to the carotid sheath and to the anterior aspect of the spine. A localization radiograph is obtained. Fragments of bone are gently removed. A high-speed burr may be used to drill out intact areas of the vertebral body and gain better access to the fracture fragments and epidural space (Figs. 19–2C and D). After complete excision of the vertebral body and decompression of the epidural space, a structural graft from the iliac crest or fibula is placed. Plating with screws often is done to stabilize the injured vertebral segment (Fig. 19–2E). Plating extends from the intact rostral to the intact caudal vertebra. A drain is used. If fixation is less than optimal, a halo device might be required postoperatively.

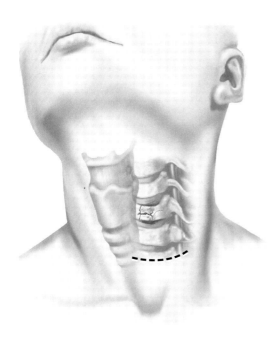

FIGURE 19–2B

A standard transverse incision is made. For more extensive injuries, an oblique incision might be appropriate.

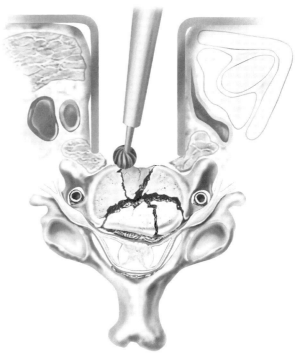

FIGURE 19-2C

Dissection is carried medial to the sternocleidomastoid, with division of several fibers of omohyoid. The carotid is taken laterally and the trachea and esophagus medially. The potential space anterior to the cervical spine is entered. After radiographic confirmation of the appropriate level, corpectomy and diskectomy are performed.

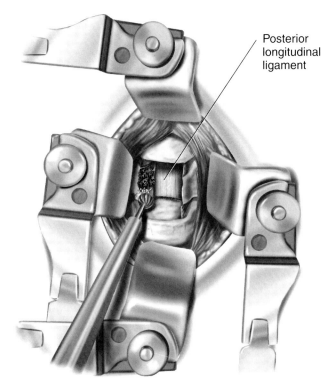

FIGURE 19-2D

After localization, corpectomy is performed. If possible, the posterior longitudinal ligament is preserved.

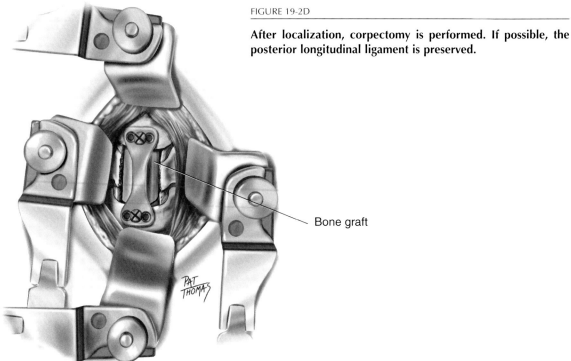

FIGURE 19-2E

After corpectomy, rostral and caudal end-plates are prepared and a structural graft is placed. Anterior plating with screws can be done.

POSTOPERATIVE CARE

When necessary, a rehabilitation program is indicated. The cervical orthosis or halo is used for 3 months to ensure osseous union.

OUTCOMES

The outcome is related directly to the severity of neurologic trauma sustained at the time of the injury. With graft and plate fixation, however, rehabilitation programs can be instituted more promptly, which might enhance functional recovery.

COMPLICATIONS

Failure of union or loss of fixation can occur, particularly with global instability. In those instances, a supplementary posterior procedure might be necessary.

20

TUMORS

- ## C$_4$ CHORDOMA EXCISION AND FUSION

- ## C$_4$ CHORDOMA EXCISION AND FUSION

SUMMARY

Tumors of the cervical spine are comparatively uncommon. Chordoma is a primary tumor of the spine that originates from residual notochord tissue. It occurs predominantly in the cephalad and caudad regions of the spine. This soft tumor grows gradually and can cause structural instability and neurologic compromise. Surgical treatment is the procedure of choice because it is relatively resistant to other forms of therapy. Recurrence of the tumor is common because complete ablation is difficult.

PRESENTATION

Patients with chordomas present with a gradual onset of neck pain and neurologic compromise. Vertebral body destruction usually is present.

NONOPERATIVE CARE

Nonoperative care is not indicated in this condition.

DIAGNOSTIC STUDIES

Plain radiographs might show nothing unusual during the early stages. CT can show the extent and nature of bony destruction and MRI the soft tissue components of the tumor and status of the neural elements.

PROCEDURE

C$_4$ CHORDOMA EXCISION AND FUSION (FIG. 20–1)

POSITIONING

Positioning is in the supine position, with the use of some form of traction on the head (Fig. 20–1A). If gross instability exists, a halo device may be placed pre-operatively.

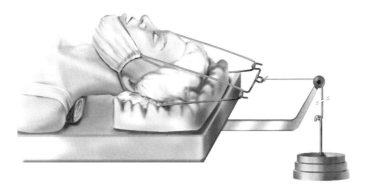

FIGURE 20–1A

TUMORS—C$_4$ CHORDOMA EXCISION AND FUSION. The patient is placed supine, with skull-tong or head-halter traction.

TECHNIQUE

This is an anterior procedure performed through a transverse or an oblique incision along the anterior border of the sternocleidomastoid (Fig. 20–1B). The side of the approach should be dictated by the extent of the disease. Exposure is obtained through an approach medial to the carotid sheath. Radiographic confirmation of the appropriate level is indicated (Fig. 20–1C). Although a true "tumor procedure" cannot be performed, an attempt should be made to remove all or as much of the tumor as possible. The tumor is often gelatinous in nature. Intraoperative pathologic stains should be obtained. Subsequent stains confirming the presence of physaliphorous cells are mandatory. After resection of the tumor and decompression of the epidural space, a structural bone graft, with or without plate fixation, is placed (Figs. 20–1D and E). The wound is closed over a drain.

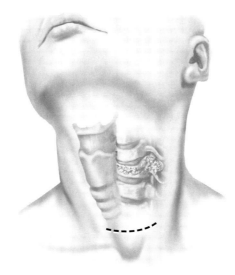

FIGURE 20–1B

A standard transverse incision is made. For more extensive injuries, an oblique incision might be appropriate.

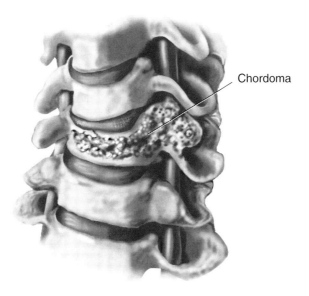

Chordoma

FIGURE 20-1C

Dissection is carried medial to the sternocleidomastoid, with division of several fibers of omohyoid. The carotid is taken laterally and the trachea and esophagus medially. The potential space anterior to the cervical spine is entered. After radiographic confirmation of the appropriate level, corpectomy and diskectomy are performed. Tumor involving the vertebral body is shown.

FIGURE 20-1D

The involved vertebral body is excised as completely as possible.

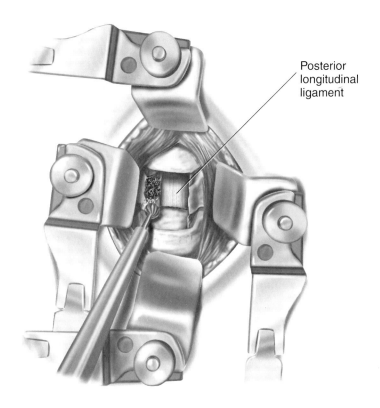

Posterior
longitudinal
ligament

FIGURE 20-1E

After resection, rostral and caudal end-plates are prepared and a structural bone graft is placed. Fixation is commonly used.

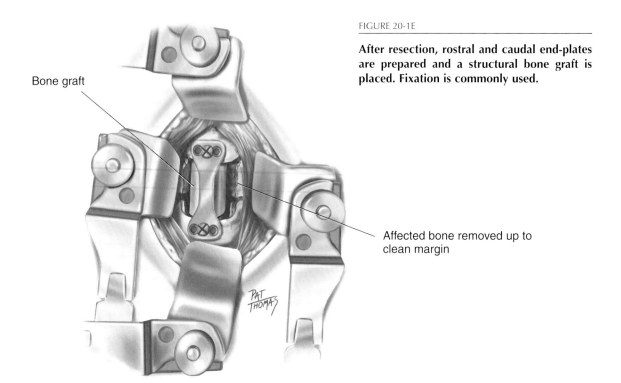

Bone graft

Affected bone removed up to
clean margin

POSTOPERATIVE CARE

Immobilization is indicated as dictated by the extent of the disease and instability present. Some patients can be managed in a rigid orthosis. Many will require a halo. Postoperative radiation may be used but is of questionable benefit. Chemotherapy has not been found to be effective.

OUTCOMES

Initial improvement in neurologic symptoms and pain should be expected. Recurrence of the tumor is common and might necessitate repeat surgery over time.

COMPLICATIONS

Loss of fixation of the instrumentation and bone graft might be encountered. Supplemental halo fixation might be necessary. Recurrent neurologic problems might be related to instability or recurrence of tumor.

21

INFECTION

- POSTERIOR DRAINAGE
  OF EPIDURAL ABSCESS
- CORPECTOMY AND STABILIZATION

• POSTERIOR DRAINAGE OF EPIDURAL ABSCESS

SUMMARY

Epidural abscess formation is relatively uncommon but can occur due to direct seeding of the epidural space or extension of infection into the epidural space from vertebral osteomyelitis. This condition is most common in immunocompromised individuals, particularly those with diabetes mellitus. In individuals with minimal symptoms, antibiotic therapy and immobilization might be adequate. In those with neural compromise but without gross osseous destruction of the spine, decompression and evacuation of the abscess is indicated.

PRESENTATION

Symptoms are usually gradual in onset. A history of an acute or subacute systemic infection followed by neurologic deterioration might be present. Fever, elevated white blood cell count, and other blood studies (e.g., elevated erythrocyte sedimentation rate) consistent with an acute inflammatory infectious process might be present.

NONOPERATIVE CARE

Positive cultures from a site of remote infection can be an indication for antibiotic therapy, rest, and immobilization if neurologic symptoms are not present. In the presence of neurologic symptoms and deterioration, surgical treatment should be considered.

DIAGNOSTIC STUDIES

Plain radiographs might show vertebral body destruction and loss of alignment of the spinal column. Soft tissue abscesses might be present. MRI is the imaging study of choice because it will show evidence of neural compression, inflammation, and abscess formation. Nuclear medicine studies can be of assistance on some occasions but are unlikely to be of benefit in individuals with acute processes and neurologic deterioration.

PROCEDURE

POSTERIOR DRAINAGE OF EPIDURAL ABSCESS (FIG. 21–1)

In individuals without major bony involvement, a limited laminectomy with abscess drainage is indicated.

POSITIONING

This procedure is performed in the prone position (Fig. 21–1A).

TECHNIQUE

A midline incision is made (Fig. 21–1B). Radiographs are used to localize the site of involvement and decompression. On occasion, gross purulence might be encountered, but on other occasions, gelatinous congealed material is present

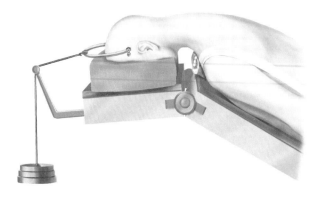

FIGURE 21–1A

INFECTION-POSTERIOR DRAINAGE OF EPIDURAL ABSCESS. The patient is positioned prone, with skull-tong traction. The neck is flexed to reduce lordosis and improve access to the spine.

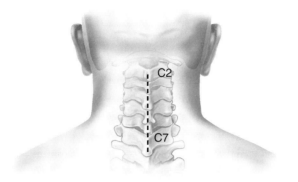

FIGURE 21–1B

A standard posterior midline incision is made.

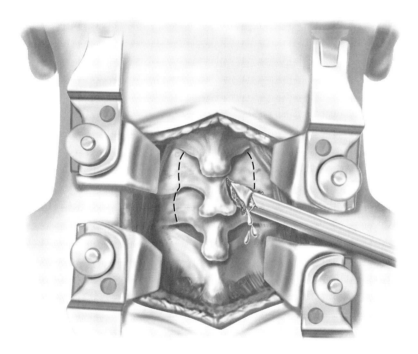

FIGURE 21-1C

A standard midline exposure is performed, with the muscles retracted laterally to the facets. Purulence may be appreciated once ligamentum flavum is opened at the involved level.

(Fig. 21–1C). It should be removed and the area thoroughly decompressed (Fig. 21–1D). Intraoperative cultures are mandatory. Antibiotic therapy should be instituted after the cultures are obtained. A drain is used. The neck is immobilized in a cervical orthosis.

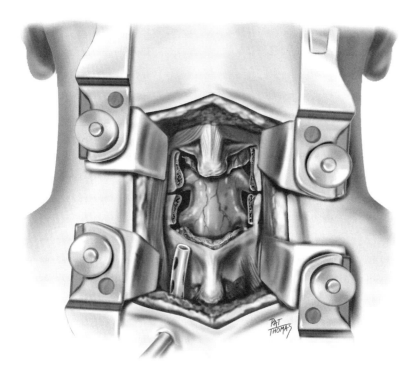

FIGURE 21-1D

Laminectomy is performed to decompress the canal. Intraoperative cultures are obtained before beginning antibiotic therapy.

POSTOPERATIVE CARE

Antibiotic therapy is continued and adjusted appropriately pending culture results. Immobilization should be maintained for at least 6 weeks and possibly longer depending on the clinical situation.

OUTCOMES

The outcome of drainage of an epidural abscess is unpredictable. In patients with acute symptoms, relief of neurologic compromise portends a better result. In patients who have had symptoms that have persisted for a more prolonged period, outcomes are less favorable.

COMPLICATIONS

Recurrent infection is more likely in cases of widespread destruction or in infection due to resistant bacterial strains. Individuals with immunocompromised states likewise may not be treated as effectively by decompressive procedures, immobilization, and antibiotic therapy. Supplemental procedures may be indicated and are dictated by the clinical situation.

• CORPECTOMY AND STABILIZATION

SUMMARY

Vertebral osteomyelitis is the most common form of infection of the spine. It can result in axial pain, fever, and, on some occasions, neurologic symptoms related to spinal collapse or epidural extension of the infection. Surgical treatment might be indicated in those situations. Anterior resection of the vertebrae involved combined with stabilization is the appropriate procedure.

PRESENTATION

Patients are frequently immunocompromised. Tuberculosis is a common pathogen in individuals who have emigrated from areas of the world where the disease is still relatively common. Diabetics are the individuals most frequently affected. Axial pain and/or neurologic symptoms are the most common causes for presentation.

NONOPERATIVE CARE

In individuals without structural collapse of the spine or neurologic compromise, a needle biopsy, appropriate antibiotic therapy, and cervical immobilization might be satisfactory. Other patients with more severe symptoms and findings should be treated operatively with debridement and structural restoration of the spine.

DIAGNOSTIC STUDIES

Plain radiographs will show evidence of osseous destruction and assess spinal alignment. Nuclear medicine scans can help in the diagnosis of occult infectious processes. CT is beneficial for assessing bony destruction. MRI is the critical imaging study because it will show evidence of abscess formation and the status of the neural elements.

PROCEDURE

CORPECTOMY AND STABILIZATION (FIG. 21–2)

POSITIONING

The operation is performed through an anterior approach, with the patient in the supine position. Halter or skull-tong traction is indicated (Fig. 21–2A).

TECHNIQUE

An anterior incision, transverse or oblique, along the anterior border of the sternocleidomastoid is indicated (Fig. 21–2B). Access to the anterior aspect of the spine

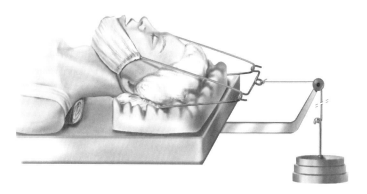

FIGURE 21–2A

CORPECTOMY AND STABILIZATION. The patient is placed supine, with a head halter or skeletal traction in place.

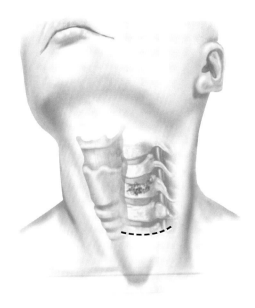

FIGURE 21–2B

A transverse or oblique incision can be used. In this case, for two-level disease, a standard transverse approach is shown.

is obtained by dissecting medial to the carotid sheath. The anterior aspect of the spine is localized and soft tissue is retracted. A localizing radiograph is obtained. Infected tissue is removed with rongeurs and a high-speed burr (Fig. 21–2C). Bone resection should be performed back to viable bleeding cancellous bone. The epidural space should be thoroughly debrided of necrotic tissue and purulence (Fig. 21–2D). Bone grafting can be used in the face of infection provided debride-

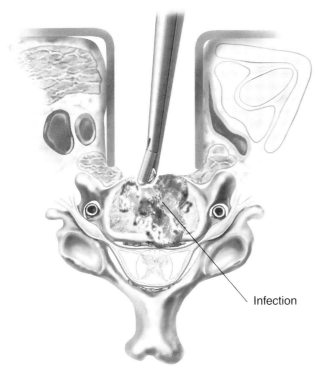

Infection

FIGURE 21-2C

Dissection is carried medial to the sternocleidomastoid, with division of several fibers of omohyoid. The carotid is taken laterally and the trachea and esophagus medially. The potential space anterior to the cervical spine is entered. After radiographic confirmation of the appropriate level, corpectomy and diskectomy are performed.

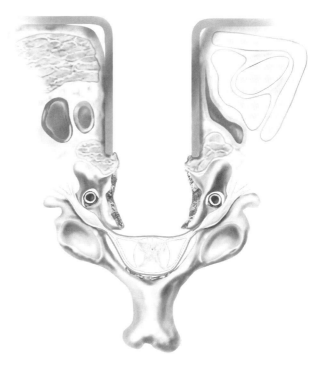

FIGURE 21-2D

All necrotic material is debrided. Resection is performed to bleeding cancellous bone; in this illustration, bone has been debrided to the posterior longitudinal ligament.

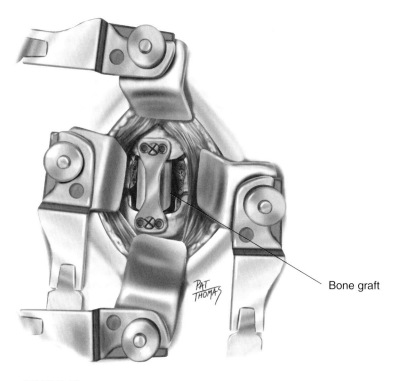

Bone graft

FIGURE 21-2E

After thorough debridement, rostral and caudal end-plates are prepared and a structural graft is placed. Primary fixation can be used after thorough debridement.

ment is complete. In most situations, instrumentation can be used (Fig. 21–2E). Where gross infection is present, bone grafting and halo fixation might be more appropriate. A drain should be used postoperatively.

POSTOPERATIVE CARE

Immobilization is generally necessary in the form of a cervical orthosis. A halo device may be used, particularly when internal fixation cannot. Appropriate antibiotic therapy is indicated for a prolonged period. An infectious disease consult might be appropriate.

OUTCOMES

As with other diseases, the outcome is related directly to the extent of preoperative problems and the ability to eradicate the disease at the time of surgery. The immune state of the patient also is important. In general, good results can be obtained with radical excision of the infectious process and appropriate antimicrobial care.

COMPLICATIONS

Recurrent infection is relatively common. Repeat surgery might be indicated, as would adjustment of antibiotic therapy.

PART IV

UPPER
CERVICAL SPINE

22

INSTABILITY

- POSTERIOR FUSION WITH WIRES AND BONE GRAFT
- TRANSARTICULAR FIXATION AND FUSION
- PRIMARY SCREW FIXATION OF THE DENS

- POSTERIOR FUSION WITH WIRES AND BONE GRAFT

SUMMARY

C_{1-2} instability usually is the result of a traumatic injury to the odontoid process or transverse ligament laxity or disruption due to injury or rheumatoid arthritis. That injury results in subluxation of the C_1 ring anteriorly or posteriorly, with real or potential spinal cord compromise at the upper cervical level. With rare exception, surgical treatment is indicated.

PRESENTATION

Patients with traumatic injuries should be assessed for upper cervical spine injury. Such injuries are relatively common in motor vehicle accidents. Individuals with rheumatoid arthritis or other inflammatory conditions can have gradual erosion of the transverse ligament, resulting in C_{1-2} instability with an intact odontoid process. Neck pain or suboccipital headache is the usual presenting symptom.

NONOPERATIVE CARE

Patients with mild instability from inflammatory or ligamentous laxity can be monitored periodically with lateral flexion–extension radiographs. Others with gross instability from ligamentous injuries or disease should be treated surgically. Individuals with odontoid fractures with gross instability can be treated with halo fixation if alignment can be maintained. A posterior fusion with wires and bone graft has been the procedure of choice for the majority of these problems when the posterior ring of C_1 is intact.

DIAGNOSTIC STUDIES

Plain radiographs will show evidence of an odontoid fracture or C_{1-2} instability. Lateral flexion–extension films might be beneficial for showing inflammatory arthritic conditions but should be avoided in traumatic conditions. MRI will assess the status of the neurologic elements.

PROCEDURE

POSTERIOR FUSION WITH WIRES AND BONE GRAFT (FIG. 22-1)

POSITIONING

This is a posterior procedure. In instances of gross instability, a halo should be applied with the patient awake preoperatively. In other situations, skull-tong traction might be adequate (Fig. 22–1A).

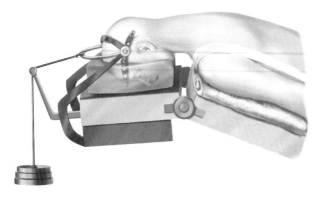

FIGURE 22–1A

INSTABILITY—POSTERIOR FUSION WITH WIRES AND BONE GRAFT. The patient is positioned prone with skull-tong traction. The neck is flexed to reduce lordosis and improve access to the spine.

TECHNIQUE

The procedure is performed through a posterior approach extending from the occiput downward (Fig. 22–1B). The posterior elements of C_1 and C_2 are identified. Radiographic confirmation of appropriate alignment is obtained. The ligamentum flavum at C_{2-3} is gently dissected free from the undersurface of C_2. A similar procedure is performed at C_{1-2} and at the occiput–C_1 level (Fig. 22–1C). A non-resorbable suture is passed ventral to C_1 and then passed ventral to C_2 (Fig. 22–1D). A cable or wire then can be easily passed beneath both posterior elements by pulling it through

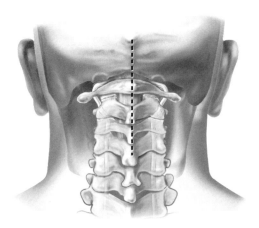

FIGURE 22–1B

A standard midline incision is made from the inion to C_{3-4}. The inion can be palpated, as can the robust spinous process of C_2.

FIGURE 22-1C

Dissection is performed in the midline (ligamentum nuchae). Muscles are dissected from the posterior aspect of C_1 and laterally to the facets at C_2 and C_3. Dissection at C_1 should not be carried more than 5 mm lateral to the midline because the vertebral artery could be injured. Care must be taken not to disturb supra- and intraspinous ligaments at C_{2-3}.

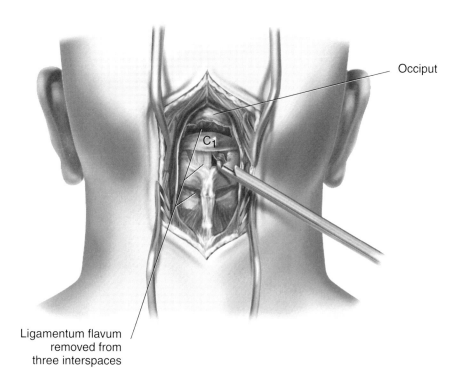

Occiput

C_1

Ligamentum flavum
removed from
three interspaces

with the suture. Blocks of bone graft obtained from the posterior iliac crest are placed over the decorticated posterior elements and the wires or cable are tightened appropriately along the posterior elements, thereby securing relatively rigid fixation (Figs. 22–1E and F). Closure is routine.

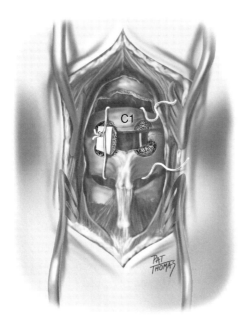

FIGURE 22-1D

The ligamentum flavum is dissected free from the undersurface of C_1 and C_2. Cables or wires are then passed from rostral to caudal under C_1 and C_2. Bone graft is placed over the decorticated posterior elements of C_{1-2}.

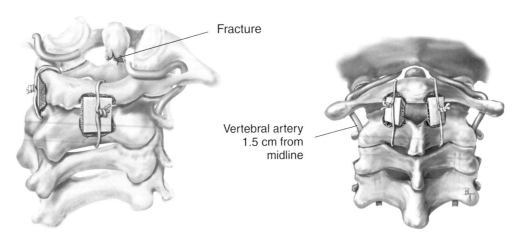

FIGURE 22-1E, F

The wires or cables are tightened to secure bone grafts between C_1 and C_2. Care must be taken to prevent anterior migration of the bone graft.

POSTOPERATIVE CARE

A rigid cervical orthosis is generally satisfactory. In individuals with rheumatoid arthritis, where osseous integrity is of concern, a supplementary halo device might be indicated.

OUTCOMES

Success rates in the vicinity of 80% should be anticipated with this procedure. In instances of nonunion, supplementary transarticular screw fixation might be necessary.

• TRANSARTICULAR FIXATION AND FUSION

SUMMARY

This procedure uses screw fixation from the posterior aspect of the elements of C_2 through the transarticular portion at the C_{1-2} junction. It can be used as a substitute for C_{1-2} wiring and fusion but more frequently is used when the posterior elements of C_1 and/or C_2 are deficient. It is technically demanding in requiring knowledge of anatomy and radiographic (fluoroscopic) control.

PRESENTATION

Because C_{1-2} instability presents as neck pain and often neurologic symptoms at the upper cervical level, patients who are candidates for this procedure might have had previous failed posterior fusions with wires and bone graft or deficiency of the posterior elements. That deficiency might be present in individuals with combined odontoid and C_1 ring fractures.

NONOPERATIVE CARE

Halo immobilization is an alternative treatment in patients with fractures. In cases with failure of previous procedures, no viable non-surgical alternatives exist.

DIAGNOSTIC STUDIES

Plain radiographs assess the overall alignment of the spine. CT assesses bony integrity and structure. MRI assesses intrinsic neurologic damage and soft tissue injury.

PROCEDURE

TRANSARTICULAR FIXATION AND FUSION (FIG. 22–2)

POSITIONING

This is a posterior procedure performed in the prone position with the neck slightly flexed. Often skull-tong traction or preoperative halo immobilization is employed (Fig. 22–2A). Biplanar fluoroscopic imaging is necessary.

TECHNIQUE

A midline approach extends from the occiput caudad (Fig. 22–2B). The C_{1-2} posterior elements are identified and exposed (Fig. 22–2C). The C_{1-2} articulation is noted. Knowledge of the anatomy of the vascular structures at these levels is mandatory. Preoperative CT determines whether or not a screw can be placed into the articular mass of C_1. If the vertebral artery is present in the area where the screw is to be placed, unilateral fixation should be used, with additional wire fixation if the posterior elements are intact. The coronal and sagittal orientations of the screw are very important, as is its length (Figs. 22–2D and E). Supplementary wiring at C_{1-2} and bone grafting can be used where appropriate. After fixation, bone graft is applied. Closure is routine.

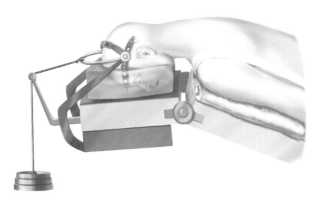

FIGURE 22–2A

TRANSARTICULAR FIXATION AND FUSION. The patient is positioned prone with skull-tong traction. The neck is flexed to reduce lordosis and improve access to the spine.

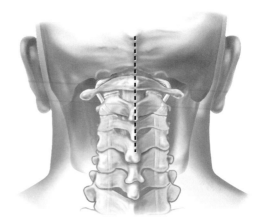

FIGURE 22–2B

A standard midline incision is made from the inion to C_{3-4}. The inion can be palpated, as can the robust spinous process of C_2.

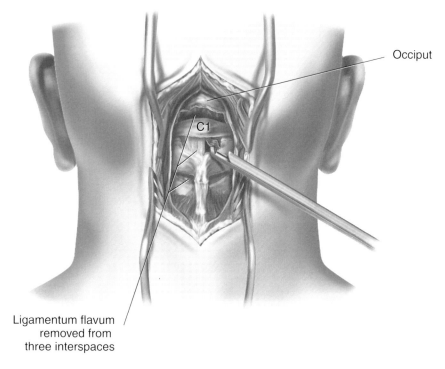

Occiput

C1

Ligamentum flavum
removed from
three interspaces

FIGURE 22-2C

Dissection is performed in the midline (ligamentum nuchae).
Muscles are dissected from the posterior aspect of C_1 and laterally to the facets at C_2 and C_3. Dissection at C_1 should not be
carried more than 5 mm lateral to the midline because the vertebral artery could be injured. Care must be taken not to disturb supra- and intraspinous ligaments at C_{2-3}.

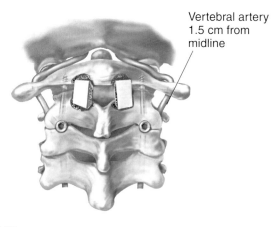

Vertebral artery
1.5 cm from
midline

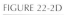

FIGURE 22-2D

The tract for the screw should begin at the inferior aspect of
the C_2 facet, with the trajectory guided by intraoperative fluoroscopy. Supplemental wiring and bone grafting can be used.

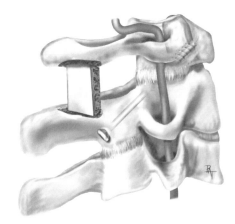

FIGURE 22-2E

Appropriate screw trajectory on the lateral view is shown.

POSTOPERATIVE CARE

No immobilization or a soft collar is indicated where fixation is adequate. Otherwise, a more rigid cervical orthosis or possible halo device can be used.

OUTCOMES

Success is generally achieved when the technical aspects of the operation have been performed appropriately.

COMPLICATIONS

The most feared complication of this procedure is injury of the vertebral artery when drilling and/or placement of the screw through the transarticular approach. If excessive bleeding is encountered, bone wax should be placed into the screw hole, the region packed, and no further attempts at screw fixation on this side should be performed. Measures should be taken to avoid this complication by careful scrutiny of the preoperative imaging studies. Cerebral insults can occur from vascular injury.

• PRIMARY SCREW FIXATION OF THE DENS

SUMMARY

Primary screw fixation of the dens is a surgical option for type II odontoid fractures of a traumatic nature. Individuals with nonunion and more chronic problems are not appropriate for this procedure. The procedure is similar to that of pinning of a hip fracture, with an attempt made to realign the odontoid process to the C_2 vertebral body and provide compression across the fracture site. This is a technically demanding operation that requires biplanar fluoroscopy.

PRESENTATION

Individuals with acute type II odontoid fractures with concomitant C_1 ring fractures in whom appropriate nonoperative alignment and halo immobilization has failed may be appropriate for this procedure. Neurologic injury is generally not present due to the nature of the injury and the amount of space available for the spinal cord at the C_{1-2} level.

NONOPERATIVE CARE

Gentle reduction and halo immobilization might be indicated in these individuals. Failure to maintain alignment might be an indication for surgery.

DIAGNOSTIC STUDIES

Plain radiographs will show the nature of the injury and gross alignment of the spine. CT is helpful to assess integrity of the C_1 arch and more specifically define the nature of the odontoid fracture.

PROCEDURE

PRIMARY SCREW FIXATION OF THE DENS (FIG. 22–3)

POSITIONING

This is an anterior procedure. Skull-tong traction or halo traction generally has been done before the performance of the procedure. The chin must be lifted out of the way anteriorly and superiorly with halter traction; a pad placed beneath the occiput helps in translational alignment of the fracture (Fig. 22–3A). Reduction should be gentle and monitored by fluoroscopic control in the anterior/posterior and lateral planes.

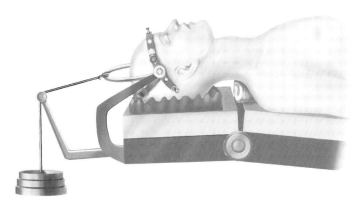

FIGURE 22–3A

PRIMARY SCREW FIXATION OF THE DENS. The patient is placed prone with skeletal traction. The neck must be extended and the chin lifted out of the way anteriorly by a combination of traction and a roll placed under the shoulders.

TECHNIQUE

The procedure is generally performed from the right side through a transverse incision at the level of C_{5-6} (Fig. 22–3B). In the initial procedures, two screws were placed. It is now deemed adequate to place one centrally located screw within the body of the dens. Screw placement is done through a central approach on the anterior aspect of the body of C_2. A cannulated screw is generally preferred. Through blunt dissection, the anterior aspect of the body of C_2 is approached (Fig. 22–3C). A notch is made in the inferoanterior margin of C_2 and the drill guide securely placed (Fig. 22–3D). Under biplanar fluoroscopic control, wire is inserted through the body of C_2 into the central portion of the odontoid process, with care to control depth. A cannulated drill bit is then placed over this guide pin and drilling performed, making sure that the guide pin does not migrate superiorly. Drilling should continue to the superior portion of the

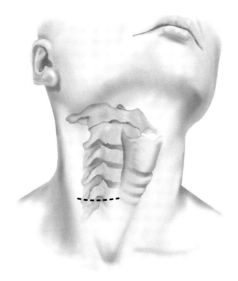

FIGURE 22–3B

A standard transverse incision is made at the level of C_{5-6}.

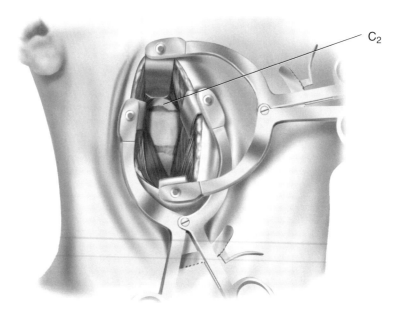

FIGURE 22-3C

Dissection is carried medial to the sternocleidomastoid, with division of several fibers of omohyoid. The carotid is taken laterally and the trachea and esophagus medially. The potential space anterior to the cervical spine is entered. After radiographic confirmation of the appropriate level, corpectomy and diskectomy are performed. Blunt dissection is then carried up to the C_{2-3} interspace. Appropriate rostral retraction is placed to maintain the exposure.

odontoid process. The screw is then inserted over the guide pin and fixation is obtained (Fig. 22–3E). The guide pin is then extracted. Flexion–extension maneuvers should be performed gently to verify the adequacy of reduction and fixation. Closure is routine.

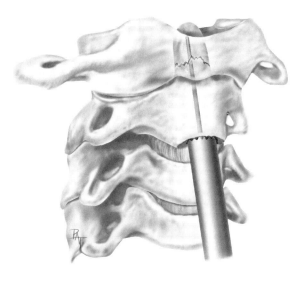

FIGURE 22-3D

Under biplanar fluoroscopic guidance, a guide wire is inserted obliquely through C_2 into the central portion of the dens. A cannulated drill bit is then placed over the guide wire and a screw of an appropriate length is placed.

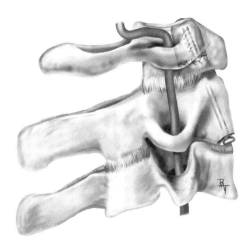

FIGURE 22-3E

Note the starting hole at the base of C_2. It is crucial that all screw threads cross the fracture site.

POSTOPERATIVE CARE

A soft collar is generally all that is required. Mobilization is immediate.

OUTCOMES

Adequate osseous integration should occur in more than 85% of cases if the reduction is adequate. Less successful outcomes are expected with displaced fractures.

COMPLICATIONS

The operation depends on technique. Soft tissue injuries during the approach range from bleeding to esophageal complications. Fixation problems might result from attempts to employ two screws in an odontoid of inadequate size. The guide pin should be monitored actively under fluoroscopy to avoid proximal migration and potential brainstem injury. Distraction fixation can result in nonunion.

INDEX

Page numbers followed by an "f" indicate figures.